Lectin-Free Cookbook

21 Day Meal Plan to Help You Get Started, Lose Weight, and Feel Great

By Clarissa Fleming

Table of Contents

Introduction

Welcome to the *Lectin-Free Cookbook: 21 Day Diet Plan To Help You Get Started, Lose Weight, and Feel Great - Forty Delicious Plant Paradox Recipes Tips and Tricks for Beginners.*

Lectin-free eating has become a way of losing weight, but it is so much more than just weight loss. It is the way that many people are finding to be beneficial for their health in either preventing or controlling certain diseases such as heart disease, diabetes, cancer, and rheumatoid arthritis.

A lectin-free diet is one that recommends the avoidance of lectins, a naturally-occurring group of carbohydrate-binding proteins. Lectin proteins are found in almost all foods. When protein is thought of, our first thought is that proteins are healthy. However, a diet that contains lectins can lead to weight gain and inflammation.

How does this happen? The lectin proteins mimic insulin and "sticks" to two places, our fat cells, and our muscle cells. This book will explain how your gut can be damaged by lectin-based foods causing irritable and chronic stomach upsets.

The lectin-free eating process, founded in 2017 by Dr. Steven Gundry, a former cardiothoracic surgeon, recommends that we eat as clean and lectin-free as possible.

The recipes are delicious and easy to make and there are even chapters for desserts and snacks. You'll find the recipes you like the most and will probably begin to create some of your own.

Every effort was made to ensure it is full of information and will make you convert to lectin-free eating. Please enjoy!

Chapter One: The Nutritional Benefits from a Lectin-Free Diet and Shopping List

For many of you who diets and looks to find healthy ways to eat and either lose or maintain your weight, you have found that many of the popular and known diets do not fulfill the results that you want. Some of you may be wondering why this happens.

Diets that are soy-free, sugar-free, gluten-free, and dairy-free are some of the many diets that have been tried and have shown some successes. However, the lectin-free diet is quite different.

The lectin-free diet, created by Dr. Steven Gundry and his findings in 2017 states that plant-based protein known as lectins should be avoided.

Dr. Gundry, a former cardiothoracic surgeon, claims that *lectins are a toxin that is hidden and lurking in what you would consider foods that are healthy.* The foods that Dr. Gundry found to have lectins are beans, nuts, potatoes, brown rice, zucchini, tomatoes, and quinoa – all staples of a plant-based diet. Gundry stated that toxins are linked to health problems that are inflammation-related such as cancer and diabetes.

Lectins – What are they?

Lectins are a type of protein that may aid the interaction of cells. These proteins also contain nitrogen, a source that plants need to grow. While most plants contain lectin, the seed is what people end up eating most often.

As a carbohydrate-binding protein found in countless plant and animal foods, lectin can be found in legumes, milk, eggs, grains, and vegetables like eggplant, potatoes, tomatoes, and peppers. Lectin can bind to cells found on the gut wall and ingested in large amounts. The gut wall can be damaged by lectin. The damage prevents nutrients from being absorbed. This can result in irritation that can cause diarrhea and vomiting.

The impact of lectins affects a person's health in many ways. The irritation of the digestive system to chronic disease are risks that lectin can create. Eating uncooked lectins may cause an upset stomach. It also has been shown that lectins cause red blood cells to cluster together and are unable to supply oxygen to the cells.

Foods that contain lectins and are eaten uncooked may cause stomach upset that's why it is dangerous to eat undercooked legumes. Phytohaemagglutin is the lectin found in red kidney beans and is the cause of red kidney bean poisoning. This is the result of eating undercooked or raw kidney beans. The FDA (United States Food and Drug Administration) has found that symptoms including severe nausea, diarrhea, and vomiting can occur by consuming just four raw kidney beans.

Cooking can break down some of the plant starch to simpler carbohydrates and cooking methods where moist heat is used can help to decrease the number of lectins in plants. Lectins attach to carbohydrates and are eliminated from the body before their effects become negative. Cooking red kidney beans in a slow cooker is not recommended because the lectins will not be eliminated due to the cooking temperature not being high enough. The ways to reduce lectins in foods include boiling, fermentation, sprouting, deseeding, pressure cooking, and peeling.

Lectins do have some positive effects. A small number of lectins can help the good bacteria that live in the digestive system. Additionally, researches propose that lectins may be helpful in identifying and diagnosing cancer. Lectins have also been studied for the possibility to slow down the degree that cancer cells multiply. They are also being looked at by researchers as potential treatments caused by viruses, bacteria, and fungi.

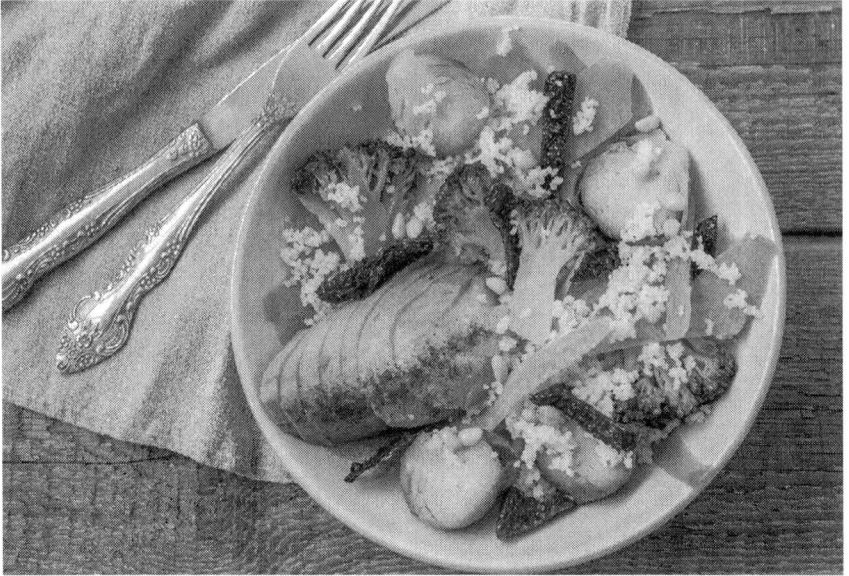

Gundry recommends discarding a large number of items from your diet to escape damage to your "leaky gut" syndrome, weight gain, and damage to the digestive system. Items recommended to be eliminated are milk, rice, beans, bread, lentils, potatoes, most nuts, cucumbers, tomatoes (unless peeled and deseeded), pumpkin seeds, chia, tofu, seeds, soy protein, and a variety of sweeteners including sugar.

A lectin-free diet is one that recommends the avoidance of lectins, a naturally-occurring group of carbohydrate-binding proteins. These proteins are found in almost all foods. When protein is thought of, particularly proteins that are naturally created, our first thought is these proteins are healthy. However, a diet that contains lectins can lead to weight gain and inflammation.

A lectins-free diet eliminates lectins from the diet in order to prevent long-term inflammation that has been linked to serious medical conditions such as heart disease, certain cancers, and depression. Lectins have also been connected to autoimmune diseases including rheumatoid arthritis, diabetes, and celiac disease.

Weight loss on a lectin-free diet is possible because when you eat high-lectin foods like wheat, it gives your body cues to store fat because the lectins do battle with your gut and your body's stored fat needs to keep battling. As stated earlier, the gut microbes, that are beneficial in absorption and our well-being by helping us to maintain a healthy weight, are depleted.

One other reason eating foods rich in lectin can contribute to excess weight is that many grains, in addition to glute, is WGA (Wheat germ agglutinin). This lectin is the most offensive lectins and has been linked in celiac and heart disease. One of WGA's most deceptive powers is its ability to act like insulin in the body, the hormone that is manufactured by the pancreas.

Insulin is released in fluctuating amounts in response to the amount of protein and sugar you eat. Your blood sugar levels are regulated by insulin by attaching to either fat cells or muscle cells, opening them up to allow glucose in. When the glucose settles in the cell and insulin detaches. The cells then have the ability to receive messages from other chemicals and hormones.

Because WGA is lectin-laden, it attaches to the same receptor sites on these cell walls that insulin does and doesn't leave, taking the places where insulin would enter, but can't because WGA is in the cells in insulin's place. WGA attaches to the fat cells making more fat from sugar that passes by. When WGA attaches to the wall of a muscle cell it prevents any sugar cells (insulin) from getting in and your muscle can't attain the fuel it needs to grow.

So, when lectins maintain a residence on nerve cells, they lack the energy they need and continually sends a message that you're hungry in order to get more fuel. The nervous system keeps sending signals that you're hungry, WGA acts like insulin which makes the fat cells grow, calorie intake rises, and your brain cells don't get the fuel they need, creating brain fog.

In order to eliminate the results of eating foods that contain lectin, avoid consuming them as part of your diet and eating only those foods that have low to no lectins in them. Additionally, the way foods are grown, prepared, or fed, such as grass-fed beef, are the foods that you should incorporate into beginning a lectin-free diet.

When you begin to understand what lectins are and the foods that contain them, you can begin a way of eating that has a positive effect on your health. Everything from brain fog, bloating to diseases such as autoimmune disease such as rheumatoid arthritis to heart disease will begin to react to a lectin-free diet. The key is identifying lectin-free foods and having a variety of anti-inflammatory foods to choose from.

Starting Your Lectin-free 21 Day Diet Program

The first thing to do when you start a diet is checking in with your medical professional. It is important to be examined and see if there would be any issues that may be negatively affected by dieting. This is a pre-requisite for any diet that you may attempt.

Once you've been given the medical approval, it's time to get your body ready for this new experience. Your body has become accustomed to eating foods high in lectin as well as sugar and your gut has had bad bugs in it for years. And now, it's time to say goodbye to all of the foods filled with lectins and rid your refrigerator and pantry shelves of all the types of foods you won't be eating any longer.

When you eat lectin-free foods, your gut can benefit by changing your diet. Your body will only take three days to begin reducing its inflammation, improve the balance of bacteria, lose a little bit of weight (which will initially be water weight), and develop a better sense of well-being.

Detox – How Does it Work?

A good way to prepare your body for your 21-day diet is by detoxing it over the first three days of your diet. This is a simple detox that will cleanse your gut, but your immune response will be stimulated.

You will discontinue ingesting all grains/pseudo grains, dairy, sugar, eggs, seeds, soy, nightshade plants, tubers, corn, roots, inflammatory oils, and farm animal proteins.

Discontinue Foods containing Lectin

The list below indicates all the foods that are laden with lectin:

- **Starches** – potatoes, rice, pasta, milk, bread, tortillas, pastry, cookies, potato chips, crackers, grain and pseudo flours, cereal, sugar, Sweet n Low, Splenda, NutraSweet, SweetOne or sunett NutraSweet, Maltodextrin, and diet drinks.

- **Vegetables** – tomatoes and cucumbers (both can be eaten if peeled and the seeds are taken out), sugar snap peas, chickpeas, peas, ripe bananas, tofu, soy, legumes, edamame, all beans including sprouts, soy protein, all lentils, and textured vegetables
'
- **Nuts & Seeds** – cashews, pumpkin, chia, peanuts, and sunflower seeds

- **Fruit& Vegetables** – ripe bananas, melons, zucchini, pumpkins, eggplants, squashes, chili peppers, bell peppers &, goji berries, and all fruits (except in-season fruit)

- **Oils** –grapeseed, cottonseed, sunflower, safflower, soy, corn peanut, canola, or vegetable oils

- **Grain or soybean-fed fish** - shellfish, lamb poultry, pork, and beef,

- **Sprouted/pseudo grains and grasses** – wheat, Kamut, oats, quinoa, whole grains, kashi, buckwheat, spelt, corn and corn products, cornstarch, corn syrup, brown rice, white rice, wheatgrass, barley grass, and popcorn

- **Cow's milk products** – a-1 Yogurt contains casein, Greek yogurt, frozen yogurts, American cheese, Ricotta, cottage cheese, and Casein protein powders

Now that you have the mindset to say no to all the foods containing lectin, it's time to purchase some of the vegetables on the shopping list. They are all lectin-free and will be part of your three-day detox.

The following is your entire shopping list beginning with your veggies:

The Lectin-Free Shopping List

Below are the foods that are recommended for a lectin-free diet:

- **Vegetables/Plant foods** - cauliflower, garden cress, bok choy, cabbage, broccoli, Brussels sprouts, garlic, spinach, asparagus, carrots, mushrooms, watercress, endive, escarole, mustard greens, leeks, artichokes, algae, kale, radicchio, kimchi, collards, celery, leeks, scallions, onions, carrots, parsley, seaweed, sea vegetables, basil, okra, dandelion greens, fennel, butter lettuce, asparagus, mizuna, purslane, algae, perilla, chives, mushrooms, cassava, yucca, baobab fruit, celery root, parsnips, rutabaga, persimmon, taro root, jicama, turnips, green mango, tiger nuts, green papaya, millet sorghum, and mint.

- **Grass-fed/finished meats** – wild game, beef, venison boar, lamb, pork, bison, elk, and prosciutto

- **Pastured poultry** – chicken, quail, turkey, goose, duck, dove and grouse

- **Plant-based meats** – veggie burger, hemp tofu, Quorn, tempeh, and Hilary's root

- **Wild caught fish** – freshwater bass, white fish, canned tuna, Alaskan salmon, shrimp, lobster, crab, scallops, oysters, calamari/squid, sardines, anchovies, mussels, and Hawaiian fish (2-4 ounces/day)

- **Starches** - green bananas, tortillas (Siete brand), bagels, bread (Bakery Paleo Wraps and made with coconut flour), coconut flakes cereal (Paleo), and green plantains

- **Eggs** – Vegan Egg or Omega-Three eggs

- **Fruit** – Berries in season and avocado

- **Flours** - almond, sesame, coconut, hazelnut, sweet potato, and cassava

- **Oils** –avocado oil, sesame oil, coconut oil, olive oil

- **Olives** – all kinds

- **Condiments** – Mustard and sea salt

- **Vinegars** – all with no sugar added

- **Herbs and seasonings** – Miso, all herbs, and seasonings. No chili pepper flakes

- **Nuts & seeds**–macadamia, walnuts, pecans, pine nuts, coconut, pistachios, coconut cream hazelnuts, hemp seeds, flaxseed, chestnuts, sesame seeds, hemp protein powder, psyllium, Brazil nuts (One-half cup/day)

- **Dairy products** – A2 milk, buffalo mozzarella (from buffalo milk), goat cheese, goat brie, goat and sheep kefir, coconut yogurt, organic heavy cream, organic cream cheese. (You may have 1-ounce cheese or 4-ounces yogurt a day)

- **Sweeteners** – Stevia, Insulin, Xylitol, and Erythritol

- **Dark chocolate** - .72% or greater

- **Ice Cream** – milk/dairy-free frozen dessert, coconut,

All vegetables provide a good supply of folate for a healthy heart and vitamin K for bone protection. They also provide prevention of inflammatory issues.

Eat as much of the vegetables as you want raw or cooked. If you have digestions problems, Irritable Bowel Syndrome (IBS), and other issues, you may want to cook the vegetables thoroughly. Frozen and fresh veggies are acceptable as long as they are organic.

You can eat small amounts of fish and pastured chicken. However, no more than two 2 to 4 ounces of each per day. The fish should be wild-caught. For portion size, a deck of cards is a good comparison to use.

The foods that you can have every day without worry are:

Avocado – Actually, you can eat the whole avocado with no ill effects. Eating an avocado can aid your skin's natural oil barrier to become more durable because of the avocado's fatty acids. This will protect your skin from the dangers of sun exposure.

Walnuts, pistachios, or macadamia nuts –These are the real nuts and can be great for your health. They support heart health, helps in regulating blood pressure, and aids in the protection against inflammation.

Don't be confused with what are nuts and what isn't. Cashews are seeds and peanuts are really legumes, both of which are full of lectins.

Extra dark chocolate (One ounce)–You can eat chocolate *every day*! YUM! Don't be shy, indulge yourself with one ounce as a snack. The benefits come from the flavonoids and antioxidants that have anti-inflammatory properties. The main ingredient is plant-derived cocoa which is where the real benefit comes from

For snacks, you can eat all the approved nuts to get you through to dinner or as many olives as you want. All are good to begin to derive the benefits of anti-inflammatory effects.

For your beverages, decaf coffee, unsweetened tea, and 8 cups of water, either sparkling or tap to quench your thirst.

As always, sleep is a wonderful healer, so try getting at least 7 to 8 hours of sleep each night and do some light exercising like stretching or light yoga.

The detox may be a bit uncomfortable, especially since you are doing away with the way you normally eat, but it will become easier. With the exception of the protein, you can eat as much as you want of the veggies and olives. Do go at your own pace and don't be hard on yourself. Remember, this is for your better health. Eventually, you'll be changing the bad to good bacteria ratio and that's a plus.

Be sure when you complete your three-day detox that you directly start the Lectin-Free Program immediately. Doing so will have you on your way to obtaining your ideal health.

A few more tips on how to adjust to the lectin-free diet:

You can stay compliant while you're out or traveling and don't have convenient access to your kitchen. Now that you're going to commit to being on the path to weight loss and better health, there are ways to keep you on track.

If you're looking for a protein bar that is lectin-free, there are a number that is acceptable as being compliant with the lectin-free diet. There are five that fall into the category of acceptable. They are MariGold, (the overall winner), Thunderbird, Larabar, Adapt, and Quest.

If an energy bar you've tried or were thinking of buying is not on this list, then it's not acceptable. The overall winner is MariGold. It meets the standards of being lectin-free with no sugar alcohols and all the good stuff – Prebiotic fiber, Organic & GMO-free, and Grass-fed whey. It even rates a high 5 Stars from Amazon.

There are nine lectin-free flavors such as Coconut Rage, Macarooned, ChocoNut, ChunkyChoco Pecan, Lemon Pie, Pure Joy, Chocolate Mint, Texas Praline, and Pecan Cinnabon. A MariGold sampler is great for a beginner. Beginning a lectin-free diet can be daunting, but this book is here to be a guide by giving you a shopping list of what you will need to purchase, a list of foods not to eat, and 40 easy and delicious recipes to create.

All the recipes are lectin-free and some of them will have you asking "are they sure?" because they're so good. Some of the recipes include burritos, chili, a decadent hot chocolate, brownie, cookies, and really great food.

You owe it to yourself and your health to begin this diet today! Once you've tried all the recipes and decide which ones are your favorites, you may even create some new recipes all your own.

A 21-Day diet menu has been included to help you plan out the next three weeks of eating lectin free. All the meals, snacks and desserts for the menu are included in this e-book with all the information you need to purchase the ingredients for the recipes to make this experience easy and enjoyable.

The menu below is an example of all the meals that can be eaten over the next 21 days. The choice is yours and you'll surely begin to lean towards a few favorites that you'll want to make and eat more of.

Some of the meals have an asterisk next to them. An explanation as to what the asterisk indicates is under the Helpful and Healthful tips section.

Have fun with this new experience. It's healthy and delicious!

Enjoy!

Lectin-Free 21 Day Diet Plan

All meal, snack and dessert recipes are included in the cookbook

Week 1

	Monday	Tuesday	Wednesday	Thursday	Friday	Saturday	Sunday
Breakfast	Ten-Minute Avocado Smoothie Bowl	Broccoli Cheddar Quiche	Ten-Minute Avocado Smoothie*	Breakfast Burrito w. Egg, Spinach & Goat Cheese	Plant Paradox Hemp Seed Protein Smoothie*	Cauliflower Cheesy Muffins*	Tempeh Bacon & Sweet Potato Breakfast Burritos w. Chipotle Crema
Lunch	Pesto & Broccoli w. Miracle Noodles	Italian Style Mustard Greens Sweet Potato Soup	Healthy Natural Wraps – Romaine Lettuce & Artichoke Spread	Leek & Cauliflower Soup	Crunchy Tuna Salad w. Avocado	Sea Vegetables Chicken Salad w. Miracle Noodles	Miso Stir Fry w. Mushrooms & Napa Cabbage
Snack	Artichoke Pesto	Classic Guacamole	Dark Chocolate Candy Crunch	Sweet Hummus w. Roasted Garlic	Walnuts, Macadamia nuts or Pine Nuts	Sweet Potato Toast	Rainbow Vegetables Oven Fries**
Dinner	Steak & Spinach Salad	Lectin Free Chili	Alaskan Salmon Cakes w. Spinach Pesto & Avocado	Wild Shrimp w. Greens & Lemon Oil	Chicken & Goat Cheese Enchiladas	Refreshing Citrus Fried Jackfruit Tacos	Five-Spice Pork Belly w. Cauliflower Rice & Broccoli Sprouts
Dessert	Rich Dark Brownies w. Large Sea Salt Flakes*	Snickerdoodle Cookies*	Classic Hot Chocolate*	Sugar-free White Chocolate*	Mint Chocolate Cookies*	Orange Cranberry Muffins*	Chocolate Raspberry Ice Cream Squares*

Week 2

	Monday	Tuesday	Wednesday	Thursday	Friday	Saturday	Sunday
Breakfast	Ten-Minute Avocado Smoothie*	Breakfast Burrito w. Egg, Spinach & Goat Cheese	Ten-Minute Avocado Smoothie Bowl	Cauliflower Cheesy Muffins*	Broccoli Cheddar Quiche	Tempeh Bacon & Sweet Potato Breakfast Burrito w. Chipotle Crema	Plant Paradox Hemp Seed Protein Smoothie
Lunch	Healthy Natural Wraps – Romaine Lettuce & Artichoke Spread	Leek & Cauliflower Soup	Crunchy Tuna Salad w. Avocado	Italian Style Mustard Greens Sweet Potato Soup	Miso Stir Fry w. Mushrooms & Napa Cabbage	Pesto & Broccoli w. Miracle Noodles	Sea Vegetable Chicken Salad w. Miracle Noodles
Snack	Dark Chocolate Candy Crunch	Sweet Hummus w. Roasted Garlic	Artichoke Pesto	Walnuts, Macadamia nuts or Pine nuts	Classic Guacamole	Rainbow Vegetables Oven Fries	Sweet Potato Toast
Dinner	Five Spice Pork Belly w. Cauliflower Rice & Broccoli Sprouts	Alaskan Salmon Cakes w. Spinach Pesto & Avocado	Chicken & Goat Cheese Enchiladas	Lectin Free Chili	Wild Shrimp w. Greens & Lemon Oil	Steak & Spinach Salad	Refreshing Citrus Fried Jackfruit Tacos
Dessert	Classic Hot Chocolate*	Sugar Free White Chocolate*	Mint Chocolate Cookies*	Rich Dark Brownies w. Large Sea Salt Flakes*	Snickerdoodle Cookies*	Chocolate Raspberry Ice Cream Squares*	Orange Cranberry Muffins*

Helpful and Healthful Tips

Repeat Week 1 for the third week. You can also mix and match the meals as you wish and what you want to eat. You can use the lunch recipes for dinner and the same for the dinner recipes. You can also create one of your own dishes if you desire.

Eating tip – Eat slowly and enjoy your meal. Don't eat and be distracted by watching TV or getting involved with your mobile phone, tablet or computer. Turn them off. Focus on your meal. Enjoy and savor every bite so you can feel full and satisfied.

Recipe preparation tip – Prepare portions of your meals ahead of time so all you have to do is pop it in the oven Some of the recipes include using cassava tortillas. Make enough for the week so they're at the ready to use.

*Meals - These can be switched off and eaten as a snack if you don't eat after-dinner dessert. The smoothies can also be made in advance to take to the job or wherever you are and can be your snack for the afternoon. If you have a refrigerator available to keep the smoothie cold, that snack will work.

Calories – don't concentrate on the calories. Instead, concentrate on the portion sizes and not falling back into old eating habits using lectin- filled foods.

Drink your water! - In the beginning of your diet, you may get mild headaches. It may be because you're dehydrated. Drink at least 64 oz. of water per day. It also helps to flush out the toxins in the body.

Print out your shopping list – make a copy of the list of accepted foods and create your weekly shopping list. This way you won't be tempted to "substitute" with any foods that are not acceptable

Breakfast! The most important meal of the day!

Most people barely have the time to sit and casually eat breakfast during a busy work week, but some of these breakfast recipes can be pre-made and refrigerated or frozen and reheated when you're on the run. And for the weekend, try some of the more relaxed recipes that you can savor during your leisurely Saturday or Sunday breakfast.

Cauliflower Cheesy Muffins

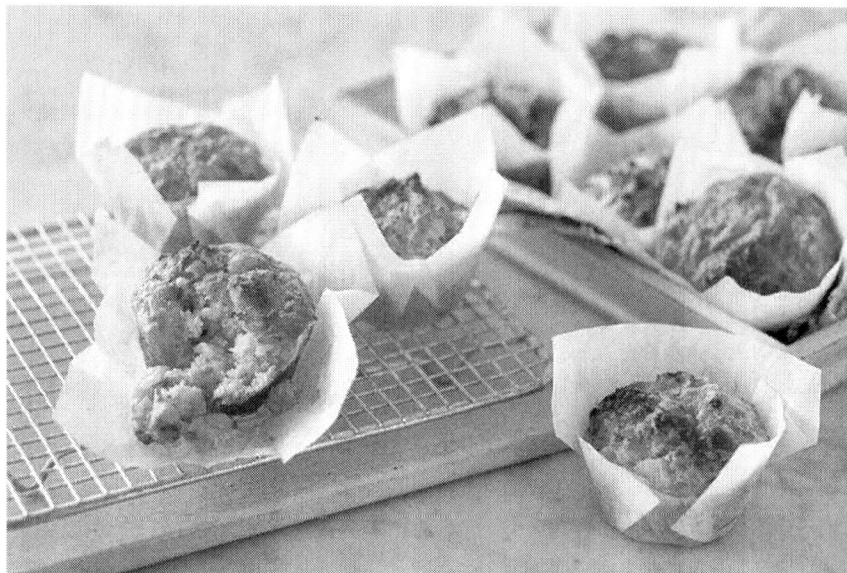

They are perfect on-the-go muffins to grab on a busy morning. They 're a sublime blend of savory cheese and egg – the perfect combo that you want in a breakfast. A dash of hot sauce gives these muffins an extra boost.

Muffins: 12
Cooking Time: Thirty Mins
Time Needed for Preparation: Ten Mins

- Three omega-3 eggs or Vegan Eggs
- Three c. cauliflower rice
- One-fourth t. garlic powder
- One-half t. sea salt - iodized
- One-fourth t. paprika
- One T. extra virgin olive oil
- One-half c Parmigiano-Reggiano grated cheese or nutritional yeast
- One-half t. dried basil
- One-fourth c. cassava flour
- One-half t. aluminum-free baking powder
- Optional – a dash of hot sauce

Preparation

1. Prepare a muffin tin with cupcake liners. Preheat the oven to Three hundred seventy-five degrees.

2. Over medium-high, in a sauté pan, heat the olive oil. Place the cauliflower rice and sea salt. Cook the cauliflower, stirring continuously for three to five mins until the cauliflower is tender.

3. Blend in the paprika, basil, and garlic powder and cook all the ingredients for an additional two mins. In a room temperature, cool after removing from heat.

4. Mix in a large-sized dish the cauliflower mixture, eggs, and cheese or nutritional yeast.

5. Whisk the baking powder and cassava flour using a small bowl.

6. Fold the dry ingredients into the cauliflower mix along with the hot sauce (optional), then portion the mixture into the muffin tins.

7. For twenty to twenty-five mins, bake until the muffins are no longer wet to the touch. Cool for 5 mins before serving.

8. Enjoy your breakfast!

Tempeh Bacon & Sweet Potato Breakfast Burritos with Chipotle Crema

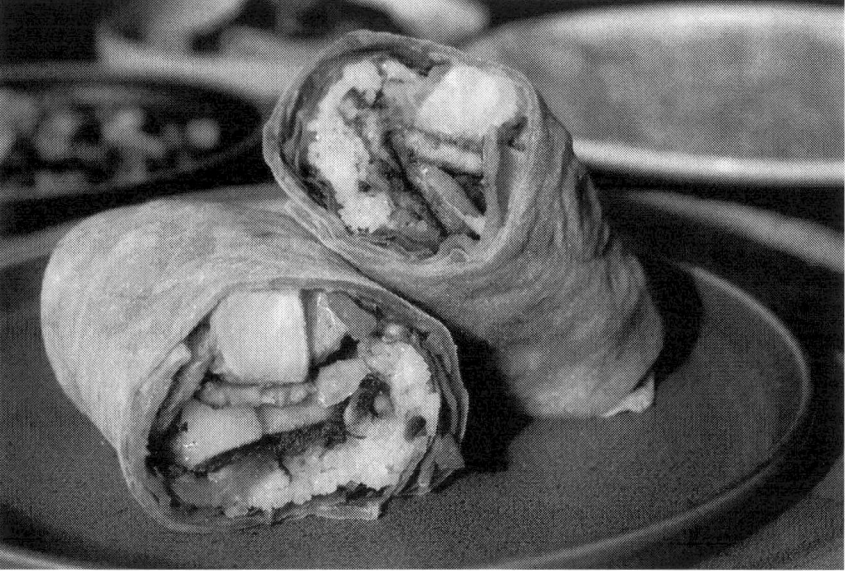

These large cassava tortillas are filled with crispy nutritional sweet potato chunks, smoky tempeh bacon & onion stir-fry, and chipotle infused sour cream.

Time Needed for Cooking and Preparation: 45 Mins
Makes: 2

Tempeh Bacon & Onion Stir-Fry

- 4 ounces tempeh, cut into thin 2-inch slices
- Water
- Two t. tamari
- Two T. olive oil
- Two t. chipotle in adobo sauce, finely chopped*
- One-half t. paprika
- One t. rice or apple cider vinegar
- One t. liquid smoke
- One-fourth t. garlic powder
- One-half medium onion, cut into small wedges
- pinch of salt
- dash of cinnamon

- 5 drops liquid stevia

Roasted Sweet Potato

- One-half large Hannah sweet potato (white sweet potato), diced
- One T. olive oil
- One T. nutritional yeast
- One-fourth t. dried oregano
- One-fourth t. paprika
- large pinch of salt

Chipotle Crema

- One-half c linked sour cream*
- One T. water
- One-half t. chipotle in adobo sauce, finely chopped*
- One-fourth t. onion powder
- pinch of salt

Assembling

- White rice or cauliflower rice
- Spring mix or baby greens
- Two large cassava tortillas

Preparation

1. Use parchment paper on lining a cookie sheet. Preheat oven to five hundred degrees Fahrenheit.
2. Toss sweet potato chunks with olive oil, nutritional yeast, paprika, oregano, and a very large pinch of salt.
3. While the oven heats up, place the tempeh into a medium-sized pan and add enough water to barely

cover the tempeh. Stir in the tamari, liquid smoke, vinegar, chipotle, & stevia. Bring to a boil.

4. Bake the sweet potato chunks until crispy on outside and tender on the inside or about 12 mins.

5. Cook until all of the water has evaporated then add in oil, a small pinch of salt, garlic powder, paprika, a dash of cinnamon, and oregano.

6. Cook – stirring a couple of times – until the tempeh and onions are lightly browned or about 6-8 mins. Put to the side.

7. Stir together water, chipotle, onion powder, sour cream, and a small pinch of salt in a small bowl.

8. Now, it's time to assemble! Place your ingredients in the center of the tortilla, positioned more towards one side than the other.

9. Lay down the ingredients in this (or any) order: a handful of spring greens, cauliflower rice, tempeh and onions, roasted sweet potatoes, chipotle crema, and a handful of spring greens

10. Fold the sides of the tortilla inward, and then fold the flap of the tortilla that's closest to the fillings over the middle then tightly roll into a burrito.

11. Repeat for the second burrito.

12. Enjoy immediately!

*It is possible for chipotles to be lectin-free friendly. Some brands contain seeds and skin of peppers while other does not. Look for chipotle in adobo sauce in a glass container as opposed to a can. Chipotle in glass containers contain no skins or seeds. If lectins are a concern and you can't find one that fits your needs, simply leave it out.

*Use linked sour cream for lectin-free

What's so great about sweet potatoes?

Sweet potatoes are an excellent source of fiber and contain a range of vitamins and minerals that include calcium, iron, vitamin C, selenium, and most of the B vitamins. They are also rich in beta-carotene, an antioxidant. Beta-carotene alters to vitamin A once it's ingested. Olive oil drizzled on a sweet potato just before serving will increase the absorption of the beneficial beta-carotene. (Shubrook, 2018)

Vitamin A – a fat-soluble vitamin present in many foods. It is important to maintain normal vision, reproduction, and the immune system as well as helps the heart, kidneys, lungs, and other organs to function properly.

Five- Minute Cassava Flour Tortillas

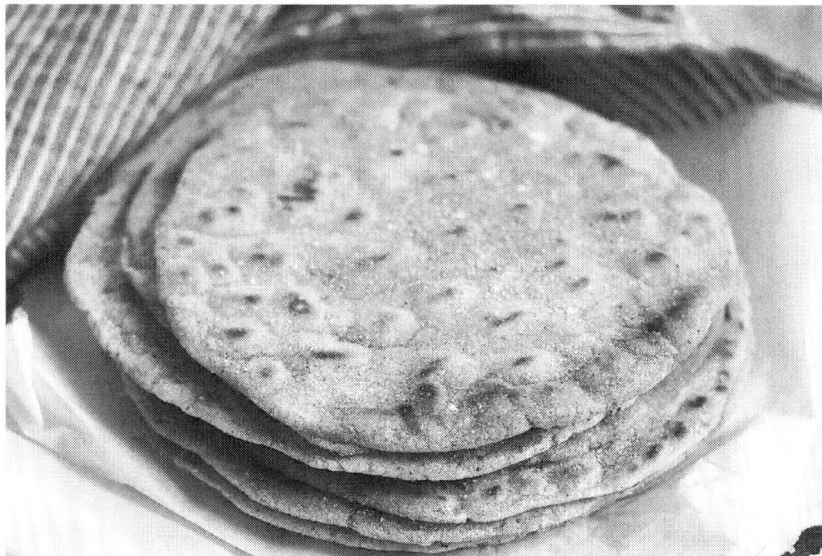

These are the easiest cassava flour tortillas. They're not complicated and are really delicious. Use them for any number of dishes.

- Two c. cassava flour – Do not use tapioca flour. Anthony's Goods brand will work much better
- One-half c of water
- One-half c olive oil
- One c coconut milk – boxed or canned
- One-Two t. sea salt – to taste
- Olive oil – for cooking
- Two t. garlic granules
- One-half t. fresh cracked pepper – to taste

Preparation

1   All the ingredients need to be combined and mixed together in a medium-sized bowl until well mixed. The dough should be smooth in consistency and not stick together.

2   Over medium/low heat, preheat a frying pan on the stove. Pour some olive oil into the pan for cooking.

3   Divide dough into ten parts, equal in size. Shape each part like a ball. Roll and pat each ball on parchment into a thin tortilla. Use a rolling pin or your hands. Sprinkle lightly with cassava flour to prevent the dough from sticking.

4   Cook one to three mins on each side until lightly browned on both sides. For a crisper tortilla, cook longer than three mins.

Cassava flour is gluten, grain, and nut-free. The plant is a staple to the million inhabitants of parts of Asia, Africa, and primarily those in South America.

Cassava flour is not poisonous. The cassava naturally contains cyanide compounds that are also found in almonds and spinach and it can be extremely toxic, however, only if the cassava roots are eaten raw. People of traditional cultures that use the cassava root as a food soak, cook, and ferment it to remove the compounds.

Breakfast Burrito with Egg, Spinach and Goat Cheese

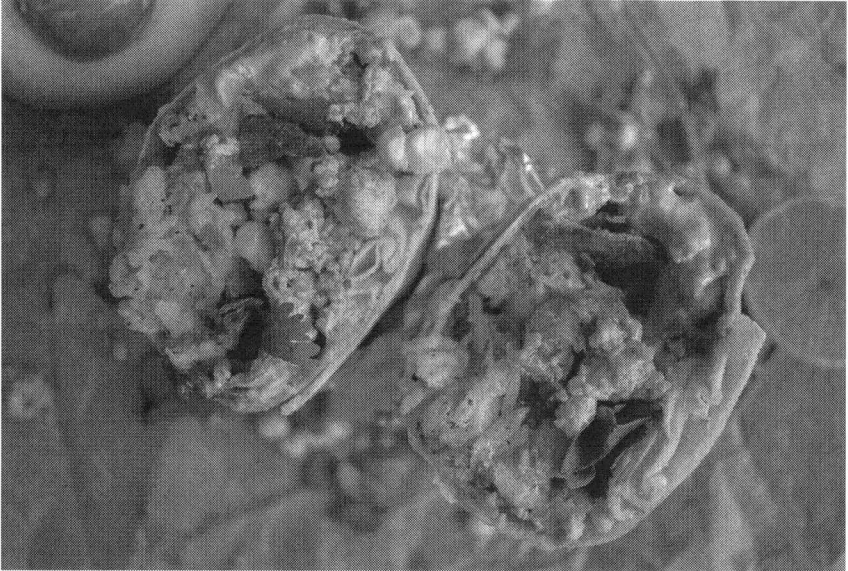

Time Needed for Preparation: Ten Mins
Overall Time Required: Fifteen Mins
Makes: 4

- Two ounces spinach, chopped
- Two sliced thin cloves of garlic
- Salt and black pepper – (sea salt)
- 6 eggs, beaten – Omega Three or VeganEgg
- 1 ounce of goat cheese – crumbled
- Two T. olive oil - extra virgin
- Eight 6 in or 8 inch cassava tortillas

Preparation

1 Use a large pan over medium heat to warm oil.

2 Add the spinach, one-half t. salt, one-fourth t. pepper, and the garlic. Cook for two-three mins until the spinach is wilted, and then spread evenly across the pan.

3   Pour the eggs over the spinach and garlic and allow them to rest for thirty seconds. Then, using a spatula, mix the eggs and spinach around the pan until set or about 3 - 4 mins.

4   Turn off the heat. Spread the goat cheese over the eggs and spinach mixture and let it soften.

5   While the cheese is softening, heat the tortillas in the microwave. IMPORTANT – **use a damp paper towel and cover the tortillas.** This will make the tortillas pliable to fold the eggs, spinach, and cheese into the tortillas.

6   Heat 4 tortillas at a time for 30 seconds each.

7   Spoon in the eggs into each tortilla and fold like a taco and serve.

This burrito recipe serves 4 and makes for a great weekend breakfast or brunch!

Ten-Minute Avocado Smoothie Bowl

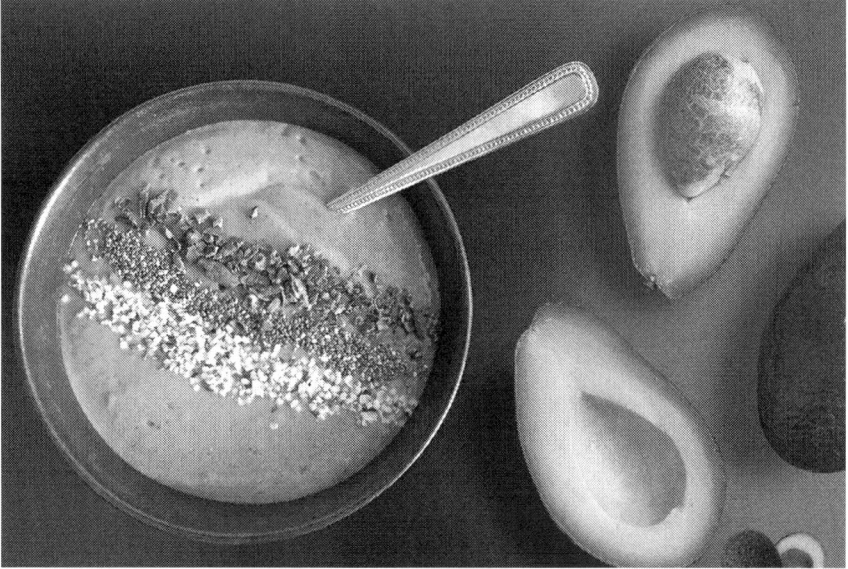

This next breakfast is a smoothie – in a bowl! Quick and easy. It can also be a midday snack. It is lectin-free and sugar-free, a different way to have a smoothie!

Time Needed for Preparation: Ten Mins
Makes: One

- Three ounces Ripe avocado meat – about One large avocado
- Three ounces (One-fourth c + Two T.) Water
- Three ounces (One-fourth c + Two T.) Full-fat coconut milk
- Three ounces of ice (6 One-inch cubes)
- One T. erythritol
- One One-half T. flax meal
- One t. matcha (optional)
- One-fourth t. liquid stevia
- One-fourth t. vanilla extract
- One T. Extra virgin olive oil (optional)*
- Medium pinch of salt

Toppings

- Toasted coconut flakes**
- Crushed Pistachios
- Fresh blueberries

Preparation

1. Using a personal-sized food processor or blender, combine all ingredients. Blend together until creamy.

2. The smoothie is intended to be thick. Pause from blending the ingredients, shake them manually, and then continue to blend again. Repeat this process until the mixture is smooth or for 1-2 mins.

3. If the mixture is too thick, add more water and blend again.

4. Transfer the mixture to a bowl and sprinkle approximately two tablespoons each of the coconut flakes, crushed pistachios, and fresh blueberry toppings over the mixture. You can add any other toppings you desire.

5. Immediate Enjoyment!

*If you wish to get some additional antioxidants into your day, add extra virgin olive oil. This breakfast meal is highly recommended. Just for fun meal, leave the oil out.

**If your coconut flakes are raw, you can make them toasted by heating the oven to three hundred fifty degrees Fahrenheit and spreading a layer of coconut flakes on a parchment-lined cookie sheet. When the oven is ready, put the cookie sheet in, and set the timer. Bake for 15 mins. Removed and use immediately, or allow them to cool. Use a container that is airtight to store in a place that is cool. They will stay ready for use for several months.

Almost everyone loves chocolate and this next decadent and refreshing smoothie is full of Omega-3s, Omega-6s, antioxidants, and prebiotic fiber that are just plain healthy.

Chocolate Super Smoothie

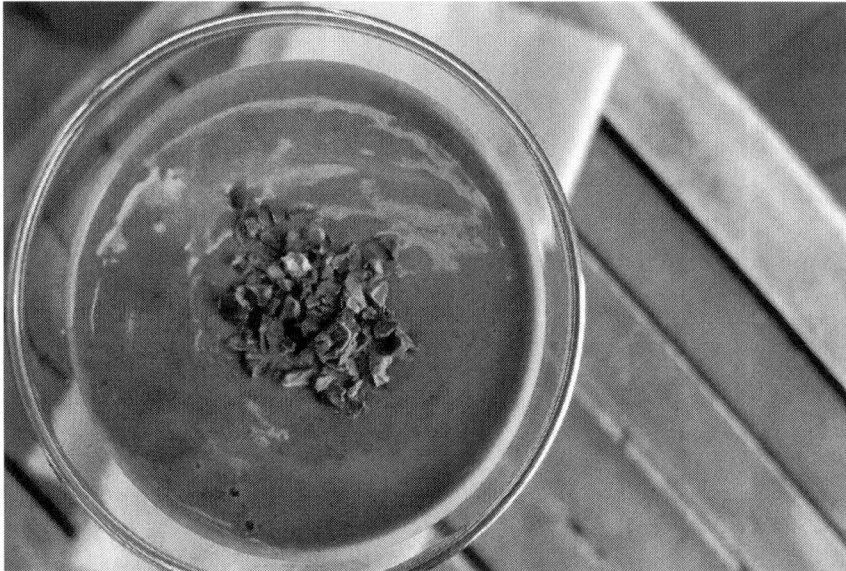

Time Needed for Preparation: 5 Mins
Serves: One meal replacement

- Three-four large ice cubes (3-4 ounces)
- small pinch of salt
- One-half t. matcha
- One-half t. stevia extract
- One T. cacao or natural cocoa powder
- One T. blanched almond butter***
- Two T. organic extra virgin olive oil**
- Two T. flax meal (use cold-milled for the preservation of fats)
- One T. green banana flour*
- One-fourth of a medium ripe avocado (about one ounce)
- 8-10 ounces water
- Two ounces full-fat coconut milk or coconut cream

Preparation

1   In a blender, place three ice cubes, 8 ounces of water, and the remaining ingredients.

2   Blend for about thirty seconds until creamy.

3   Add an extra two ounces of water if the mixture is too thick. To make it colder, add an additional ice cube.

4   Immediately enjoy or it can be stored up to twelve hours in the refrigerator or a thermal cup.

*You may use a tablespoon of pressure-cooked chickpeas like Eden Beans in place of green banana flour to be used for resistant starch.

**A really important note that can't be stressed enough: It will taste better and have more antioxidant if you use a higher quality olive oil. Imported oils from Spain or Italy are extra good oils.

***You may leave out the blanched almond butter if you don't have it. You can use coconut butter, pecan butter, and walnut butter as a replacement.

Plant Paradox Hemp Seed Protein Smoothie

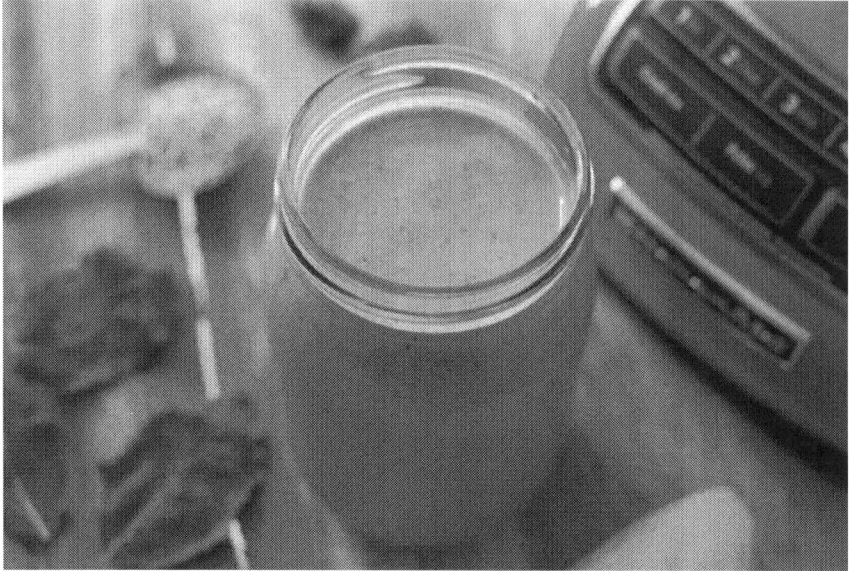

Time Needed for Preparation: Ten Mins

Makes: One

- One c organic baby kale leaves
- Two c organic baby spinach leaves
- Two Droppers of liquid stevia (Sweet Leaf Sweet Drops Sweetener recommended)
- Two T. Nutiva Hemp Protein
- One c of ice
- Two c of filtered tap water
-

Preparation

1 Blend in a high-powered blender for 30 seconds.

2 Add in a green banana and blend for another 30 seconds. Green banana is allowed as it has not increased its sugar content. It's good for your gut because it's resistant starch.

3 Add in one-fourth c ice cubes and crush the ice.

4   Pour into a cup and enjoy!

Broccoli Cheddar Quiche

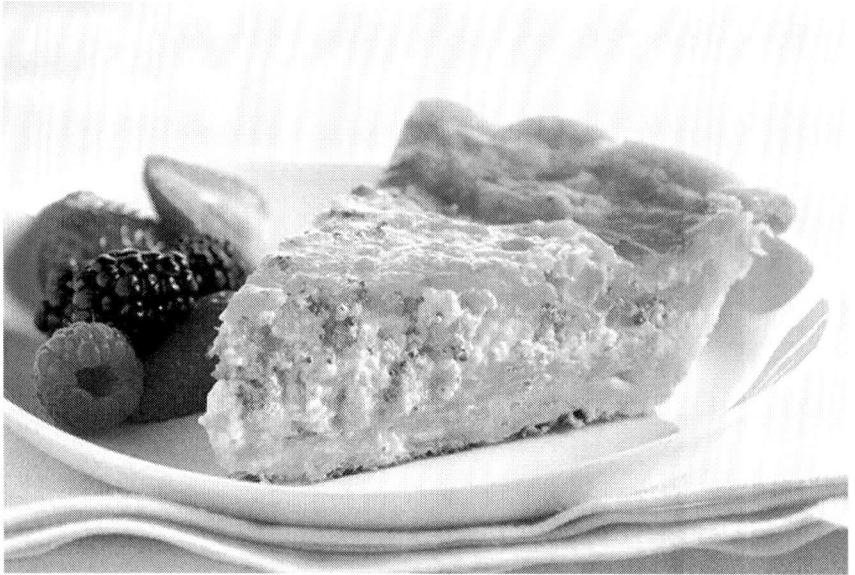

This quiche is a breakfast that you can pre-make and eat when you want to have a breakfast slice ready to warm up during your busy week. This quiche is simple to make. You can bake the crust and prepare the ingredients the night before. The next morning, you can bake the rest of the ingredients.

Time Needed for Preparation: Twenty Mins
Time Needed for Cooking Fifty Mins
Inactive: One Hr.
Makes: 4-6

Crust Ingredients

- One omega-3 or pastured egg or Vegan Egg
- One c coconut oil
- One-half c finely chopped toasted macadamia nuts
- One one-fourth c coconut flour

Ingredients for the filling

- Omega-Three pastured eggs or Vegan Egg
- 2/3 c unsweetened coconut cream
- Two c broccoli florets (small pieces)
- One t. iodized sale
- One-fourth t. nutmeg
- One-half c nutritional yeast OR one c shredded goat's milk cheddar cheese

Preparation

1 Use an 8-inch pie tin and spray with olive oil. Ensure your oven is pre-heated to four hundred degrees Fahrenheit.

2 Make the crust by putting in the coconut flour, coconut oil, macadamia nuts, and egg and pulse them in a food processor until the mixture begins to blend. Add one teaspoon of water at a time if the mixture is too dry until the mixture becomes consistent. The mixture will be like a graham cracker crust, somewhat crumbly.

3 Once the dough is made in the food processor, remove it and press into plastic wrap. Place in the refrigerator for one hour.

4 When ready to bake the crust, press the dough into the pie tin. Use your fingers to press the dough into place. Bake for ten mins, then set to the side and let it cool. Lower the oven temperature to Three hundred fifty degrees Fahrenheit.

5 Take the broccoli and steam for two to three mins. Drain and set aside.

6   Stir together the eggs, nutmeg, coconut cream, and salt, and mix well.

7   Put the crust on a sheet tray in the event of overflowing while baking. At the bottom of the crust, sprinkle nutritional yeast or cheddar cheese. Add the broccoli. Pour the egg mixture over the top.

8   Bake at three hundred and fifty degrees Fahrenheit for 35 to 40 mins. Let the quiche cool for a few mins before serving.

9   Breakfast at its finest!

Lunch, the break we need from a busy morning. The recipes in this chapter can be pre-made the night before and taken to work to enjoy the next day.

Easy to make lunch recipes that will make lunchtime a special treat!

Crunchy Tuna Salad with Avocado

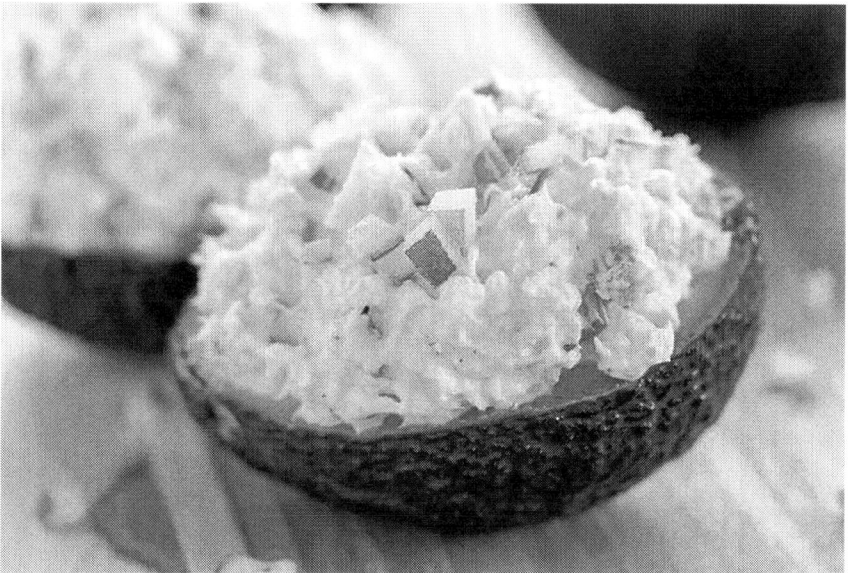

Time Needed for Preparation Ten Mins
Makes: One-Two

- 3-4 ounces of canned tuna in water or water with salt
- One long celery rib
- One-half avocado
- One small or medium carrot
- One small red onion (or a medium one, halved)
- Two T. avocado mayonnaise
- A small handful of dry-cured Beldi olives, chopped or any other black olives

- extra virgin olive oil, as much as you want/like
- salt and pepper
- lime or lemon juice

For Serving:

- Green plantain chips (or any compliant crackers or chips)
- Romaine or endives lettuce boats

Preparation

1. Chop all the veggies in small cubes

2. Mix the tuna, along with its juices with all the veggies, avocado, and olives. Add the mayo and extra virgin olive oil. Season to taste.

3. Eat with crackers/chips and romaine lettuce or endive boats.

Italian Style Mustard Greens and Sweet Potato Soup

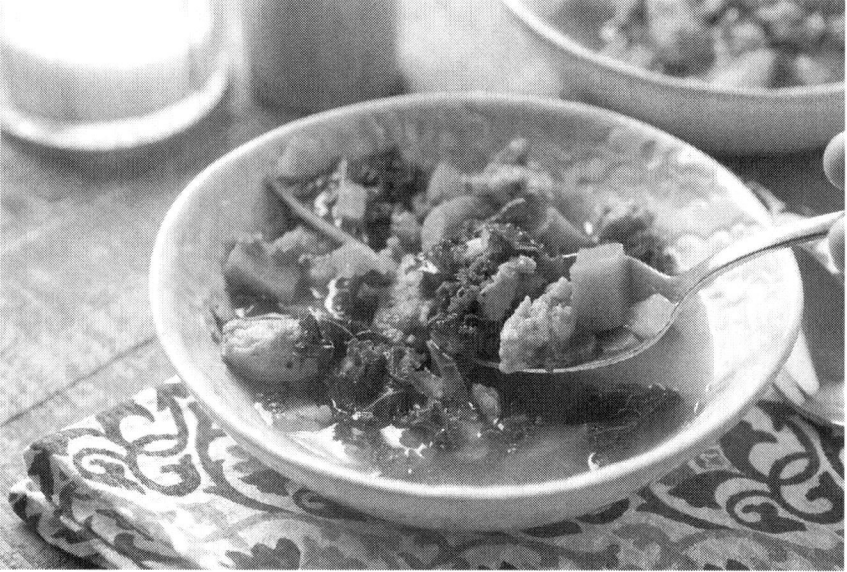

Time Needed for Preparation: Twenty Mins
Time Needed for Cooking: Forty Mins
Makes: 4-6

- Two T chicken or vegetable stock (homemade or store bought, plant paradox compliant)
- One big finely chopped celery rib
- One finely chopped medium carrot
- Medium finely chopped yellow onion
- One big bunch of mustard greens (ribs and leaves), finely chopped
- One small to medium sweet potato (you can use any color), cut in small to medium cubes
- Two garlic cloves, smashed and chopped
- One small daikon radish (optional), finely chopped
- extra virgin olive oil
- A few slices of Prosciutto di Parma. Use about 5, but you can add more or less, sliced
- shavings of Parmigiano Reggiano for serving
- lemon juice and lemon wedges
- salt and pepper

41

Preparation

1. Wash and prepare all the veggies.

2. Using a large pan, place over medium heat and add extra-virgin olive oil.

3. Toss in the finely chopped onions, daikon if using, celery, and carrots. Sauté until the vegetables soften and become very fragrant or approximately ten mins.

4. Add the prosciutto and garlic. Cook for few more mins. Then stir in the cubed sweet potatoes. Stir regularly for about 5 mins.

5. Incorporate the chopped mustard greens, stir, and cook a few more mins until the potatoes are cooked and all the greens are wilted.

6. Add everything to the stock pot and cook until boiling. Add the lemon juice, salt, and pepper.

7. Serve with Parmigiano Reggiano.

Sea Vegetables Chicken Salad with Miracle Noodles

Here's a lectin-free salad that you can enjoy for lunch or for dinner. This is an easy to make a salad that is full of nutrients and delicious. It is exquisitely flavorful. Lunchtime at its best!

Time Needed for Cooking: Fifteen Mins

Time Needed for Preparation: Fifteen Mins

Makes: Two

- One pack Sea Tangle Mixed Sea Vegetables. Rinse and de-salt per the instructions on the package
- One pack Miracle Noodles Angel Hair or other shirataki products prepared per the instructions. This is the only ingredient that will be cooked
- Two-Three medium chicken nuggets previously prepared or few slices of cooked chicken breast
- Two c of romaine lettuce, chopped
- One avocado, diced
- Two c of baby spinach

The Dressing

- One piece fresh ginger thumb size, grated
- Four T. coconut aminos
- Four T. apple cider vinegar
- salt and pepper
- One garlic clove, grated

Preparation

1 Prepare the noodles as per the pack instructions. It will take about 15 mins (rinse, boil, dry)

2 Prepare the seaweed as per the pack instructions (rinse and let dry).

3 Make the dressing by mixing all the ingredients.

4 Split the noodles in two and add to two serving bowls. Split the remaining ingredients in two. Add to the noodles.

5 Add the chicken nuggets or chicken breast if you use.

6 Add the dressing, mix well, and taste. Add more aminos and vinegar if needed.

The salad makes two main dish salad portions so you can cut the quantities in half if you only make one. Mix all the ingredients and split into two serving bowls afterward if it's easier. Feel free to add some extra virgin olive oil across the top if you desire.

Leek and Cauliflower Soup

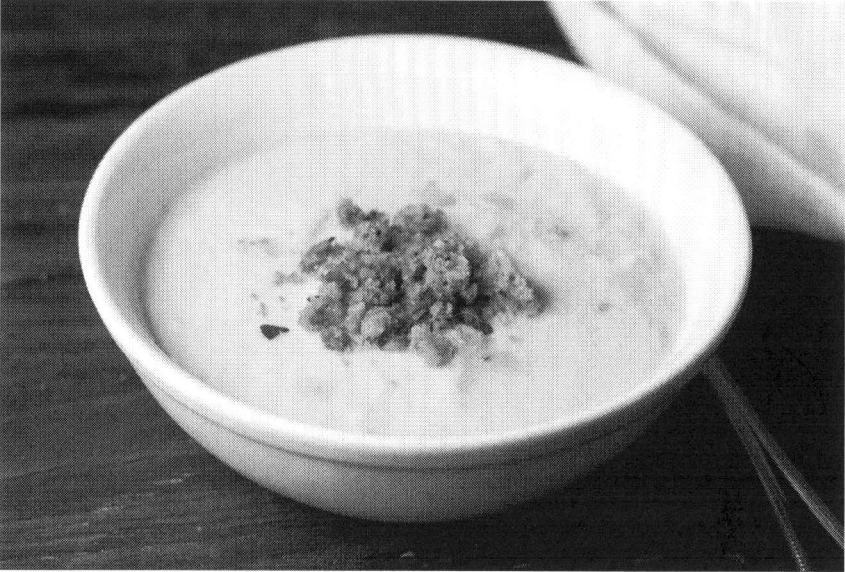

Leek and cauliflower soup mimics the leek and potato soup. Cauliflower is an amazing vegetable and is such a great substitute for potatoes in this recipe and many others.

Time Needed for Preparation: Twenty Mins
Time Needed for Cooking: One Hr.
Makes: 4-6

- For garnish: chopped chives or thyme
- One-fourth c grated Parmesan cheese – optional
- Two quarts salt-free chicken or vegetable stock
- One bay leaf
- Two t. coarse black pepper
- One-half t. nutmeg
- Three T. extra virgin olive oil
- One t. fine iodized sea salt
- One large head cauliflower – cut into two-inch florets
- Three cloves minced garlic
- Two celery stalks – diced
- One lb. Leeks – cleaned and chopped

Preparation

1. Over medium heat, place a large pot and heat the olive oil. Add leeks, celery, garlic, and cauliflower as well as the salt, pepper, and nutmeg. Sauté stirring regularly until leeks begin to wilt.

2. Add the bay leaf, the vegetable or chicken stock, and, if using, Parmesan cheese. Cover the pot and cook for an additional 35-45 mins until the cauliflower is very tender.

3. Remove the bay leaf. Use either a stick blender and blend directly in the pot or transfer to a regular bowl. Transfer a few batches at a time so you don't overfill the blender.

4. Once the entire mixture is pureed, place the soup back into the pot, and cook for an additional ten-fifteen mins.

5. Serve with chopped herbs as a garnish and additional parmesan if desired.

Pesto & Broccoli with Miracle Noodles

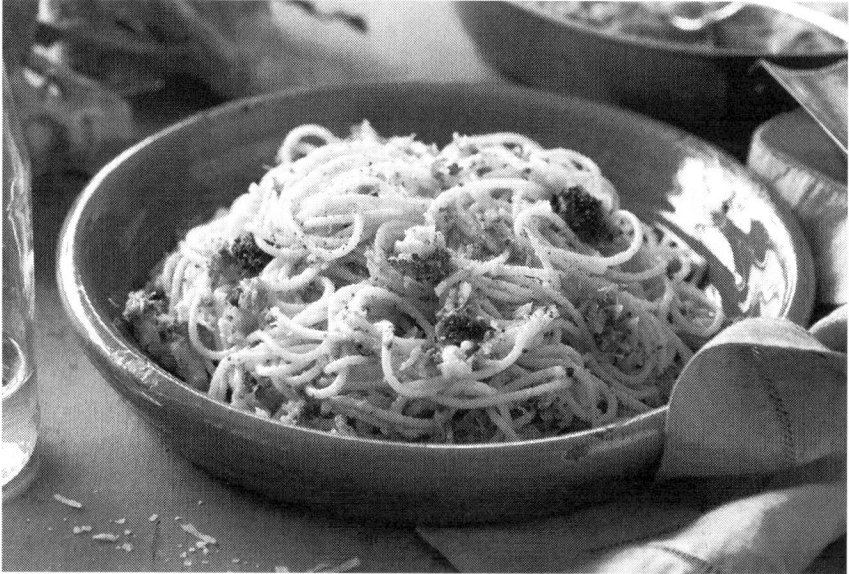

This is an easy lunch recipe that can be packed up and taken to school or work.
It has four simple ingredients that cooks in one pan.

Time Needed for Preparation: Ten mins
Serves: One

- Broccoli florets
- Extra virgin olive oil
- Miracle noodles (shirataki noodles)
  https://www.miraclenoodle.com
- Basil Pesto*

Directions

1   Heat a large skillet and cook all ingredients for less than ten mins.

*see the next recipe for Basil Pesto

Basil Pesto Recipe

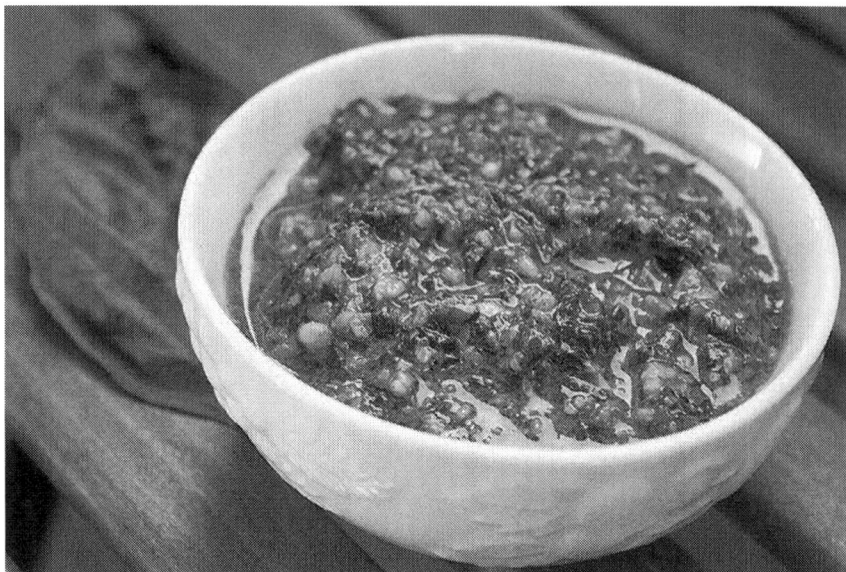

Simple yet powerful. Basil is one of the most medicinal foods that bursts with vitamins A, C, and K, potassium, Iron, and calcium.

Combined with olive oil, extra virgin being one of the best superfoods, brings a supply of antioxidants, numerous essential vitamins and minerals, and a good dose of good fats.

Time Needed for Preparation: Ten mins

- One-third c toasted pine nuts
- Two c basil leaves
- Two cloves garlic
- One-half c extra virgin olive oil
- One-half c freshly grated parmesan
- Sea salt

Preparation

1   Put the ingredients and a small portion of the olive oil into a blender and pulse until they are mixed well.

2   Stream in the remaining olive oil while the blender is at a low speed. Once it reaches a consistency that you're happy with, you've got Pesto!

Olive Oil has health benefits supported by scientific research. It is rich in healthy monounsaturated fats. It contains massive amounts of antioxidants as well as strong anti-inflammatory properties. Olive oil may help to protect against heart disease and helps prevents strokes.

Healthy Natural Wraps – Romaine Lettuce and Artichoke Spread

Romaine Lettuce – nutritionally dense of all the lettuces. They are crunchy, sturdy, and delicious. For wraps use the hearts for the artichoke spread.

Time Needed for Preparation: 15 Mins
Makes: 4

Artichoke Spread

- One jar artichokes in water and salt – Ten ounces
- One small clove of garlic
- Three T.s avocado mayonnaise
- Three T. red onion – soaked in iced water and finely chopped
- One-fourth t. lemon
- Sea salt flakes and pepper
- One T. extra virgin olive oil
- Two anchovies fillets – finely chopped

Preparation

1 Rinse and drain well the artichokes. Remove as much water as possible by squeezing the leaves in a towel.

2 In a food processor, add the artichokes and mix until well-chopped. Scrape the walls as the chopped artichoke may stick to the processor's walls.

3 Add the mayonnaise, garlic, chopped onion, chopped anchovies, garlic, and lemon, and mix in the processor again. Add some of the extra virgin oil while the processor is running.

4   Add some of the remaining oil on top of the mix at the end. Taste for the possible addition of salt and pepper, although mayonnaise and anchovies may supply enough to the spread.

5   Spread on Romaine lettuce. Roll up the lettuce and enjoy.

Miso Stir Fry with Mushrooms and Napa Cabbage

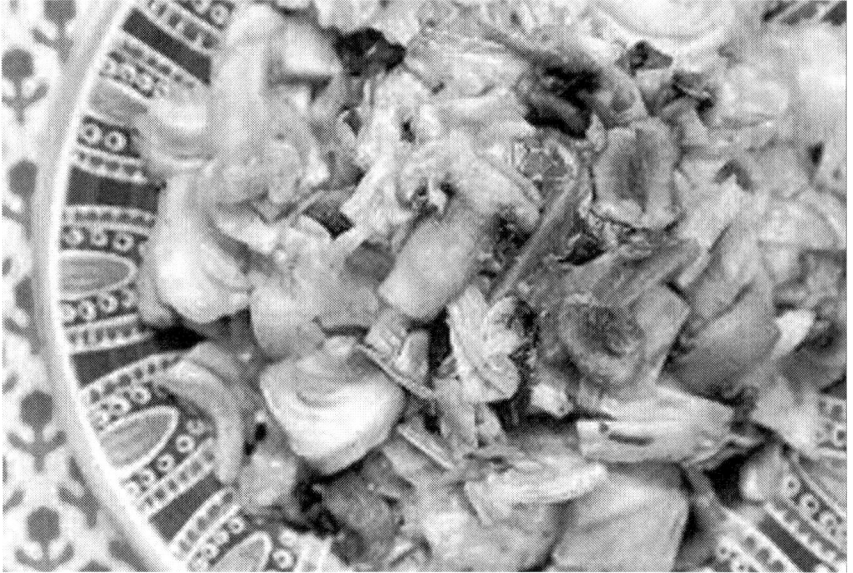

This is the perfect way to continue to incorporate eating veggies and doing so creatively.

Time Needed for Preparation: Fifteen mins
Time Needed for Cooking: Twenty Mins
Makes: Two

- 8 ounces mixed trumpet royale, forest nameko, and brown clamshell mushrooms
- 4 stems of green onion – diagonally sliced
- One-half large Napa cabbage – sliced into bite-size pieces
- One T. rice cooking wine
- Two T. Miso paste
- Two T. coconut aminos
- One T. fresh ginger – grated
- Avocado for frying

Preparation

1 Combine the rice cooking wine, miso paste, and coconut aminos

2 In a stainless steel skillet, add avocado oil and mushrooms. Saute´ until fragrant and golden over medium heat.

3 Remove the mushrooms from the skillet. Add more oil to the pan and add the ginger and Napa cabbage. Stir the ginger and cabbage for a few mins until the greenish part of the cabbage is wilted, but not overcooked.

4 Place again in the skillet the mushrooms as well as the sauce. Cook and stir for a few mins more. Add green onions.

5 Add to bowls and serve.

Refreshing Citrus Fried Jackfruit Tacos

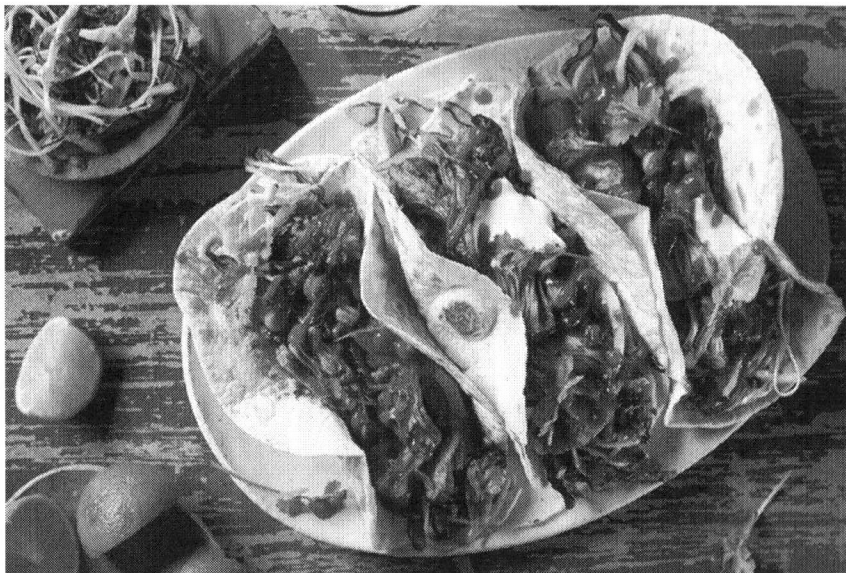

This is a Plant Paradox friendly taco that makes for a tasty dinner. It's a blend of crispy cod, jackfruit nuggets, a lime-infused beet slaw served on cassava tortillas and surrounded by lime wedges and thinly sliced avocado! This is a yum if there ever was one!

Prep and Time Needed for Cooking: One Hour
Makes: 4-6 tacos

Jackfruit Nuggets

- 7 ounces unseasoned jackfruit pieces
- Two T. tapioca or arrowroot starch
- One-half t. salt
- 1/8 t. cayenne powder
- One-half c (64 g) cassava flour
- 4-4.5 ounces sparkling water

- One-half t. baking soda
- 14 fl. ounces. refined coconut oil

Lime-Infused Beet Slaw

- Two ounces matchstick-cut beets (about One-half small beet)
- Two ounces thinly shredded green cabbage (approx. 1 /8 a small head)
- One-fourth t. salt
- One T. erythritol
- One T. sesame oil
- One T. lime juice
- one lime zest finely grated*

Orange Sweet & Sour Sauce

- Two ounces (One-fourth c) water
- Two ounces (One-fourth) ketchup (use homemade for sugar-free version)*
- One ounce (Two T.) rice vinegar
- One ounce (Two T.) erythritol
- 0.5 ounces (One T.) tamari
- One-half T. tapioca or arrowroot starch
- One T. orange zest, finely grated*

Serving

- 4-6 cassava tortillas
- Lime wedges
- Fresh cilantro
- Avocado thinly sliced

Preparation

1. **Red Beet Slaw** – In a medium mixing bowl, whisk the lime juice, sesame oil, lime zest, salt, and erythritol. Toss the matchstick cut beets and shredded cabbage

with the dressing until thoroughly coated. Place in the refrigerator for 30 mins. Cover with plastic wrap.

2. ***Sweet & Sour Sauce*** – Using a personal sized blender or a mason jar with a fitted lid, combine all the sweet & sour ingredients, blending or vigorously shake to blend.

3. Heating a small pot using medium heat, transfer all the sweet & sour ingredients. Boil and stir the sauce until it thickens. Take off from the stove and set to the side. When ready for use, reheat before serving over low heat.

4. ***Jackfruit*** – In a bowl, place jackfruit pieces. Use a separate bowl for the tapioca or arrowroot.

5. Whisk the cassava flour, baking soda, salt, cayenne pepper in a third bowl. Whisk in 4 ounces sparkling water.

6. Whisk the 4 ounces of sparkling water to the third bowl. The batter should be thick enough to stick to the jackfruit, yet thin enough that it moves freely around the bowl. If the batter is still too thick, add an additional 0.5 ounces (One T.) more of the sparkling water

7. Place all of the refined coconut oil in a medium-sized pot (the heavier the pot, the better for temperature control). Heat over medium heat and until temperature reaches three hundred fifty degrees Fahrenheit or until a wooden spoon is inserted upside down into the oil and the oil forms bubbles around the spoon's handle. (see photo)

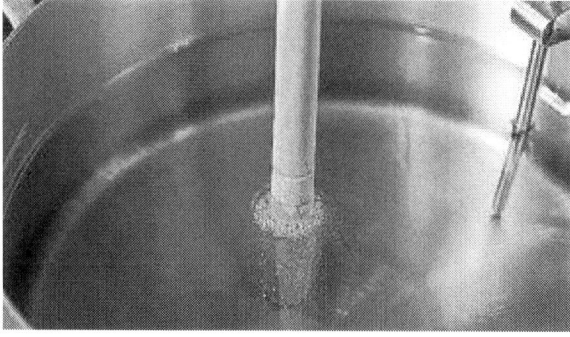

Testing the heat with the wooden spoon handle

8. While oil is heating, set up oil drain rig by inverting a
   cookie sheet onto a counter. Put a layer of paper
   towels on the cookie sheet then invert the cooling rack
   on top of that. (see photo)

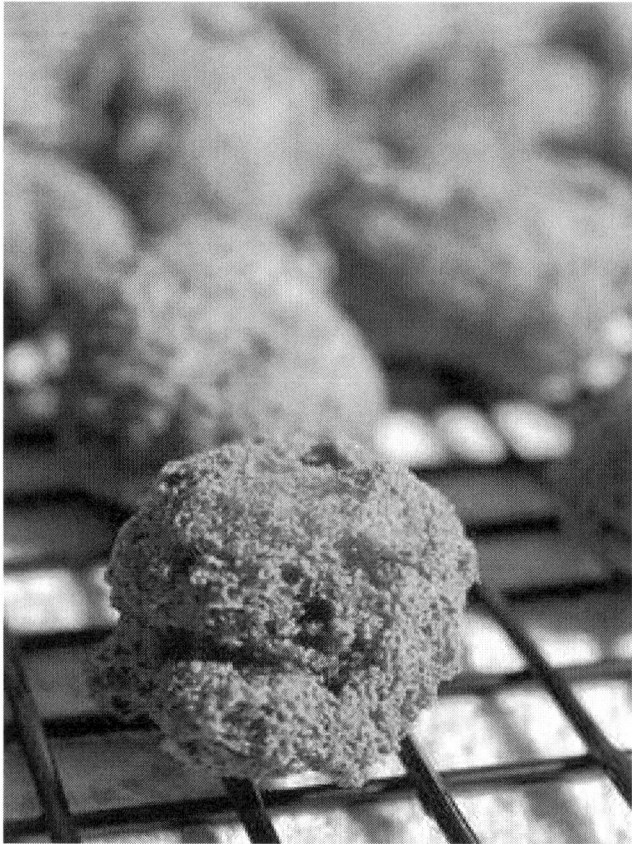

Jackfruit draining Fried Jackfruit

9. Roll a piece of jack fruit around in the tapioca or arrowroot starch, shake off excess, then dip in the batter made with sparkling water. Gently place in the oil allowing the lower portion to fry before totally immersing it into the oil. This will prevent it to stick to the bottom of the post.

10. Fry one or two pieces at a time until nuggets are golden brown and crispy, stirring them around as you go. Fry for about 45 seconds per nugget.

11. Repeat steps 8 and 9 until all jackfruit is battered and fried. Keep warm and crispy by removing the paper towels from the draining rig, Place the baking sheet right side up. Place the cooling rack back on top. Set in

a two hundred fifty degrees Fahrenheit oven for 45 mins.

12. Assemble your tacos with tortilla, red beet slaw, jackfruit, avocado, cilantro, sweet & sour sauce, and a squeeze of lime. Enjoy while fresh. Fried food is never good reincarnated.

Five-Spice Pork Belly with Cauliflower Rice and Broccoli Sprouts

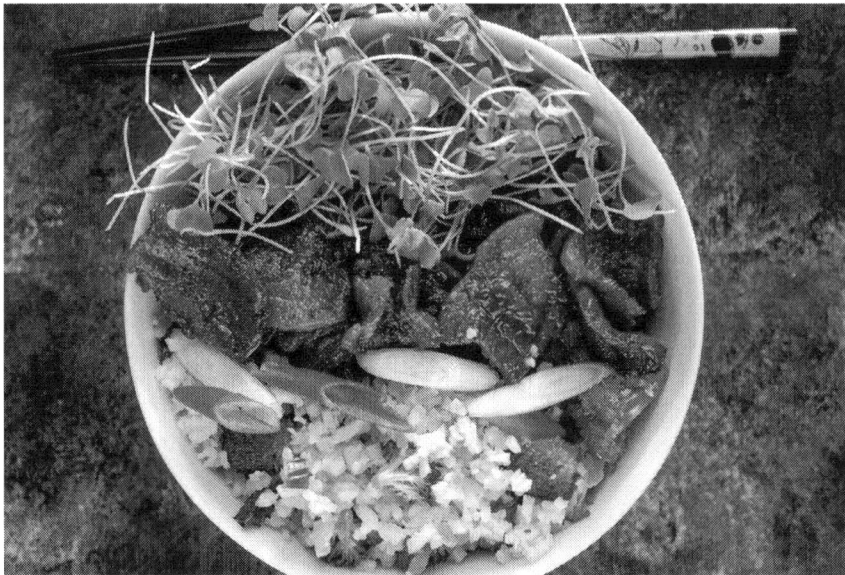

Time Needed for Preparation: Ten Minute
Time Needed for Cooking: One hr. Ten Mins
Makes: Two-Three

- One lb pork belly cut in bite-size pieces (pasture-raised)
- One c of roughly chopped red onion
- Three peeled and smashed garlic cloves
- One and one-half T. Chinese cooking wine (Mirin)
- One t. Chinese five-spice mix
- One-fourth c coconut aminos
- Two springs of green onion, finely sliced
- ¾ c filtered water
- Two t. monk fruit granulated sweetener (Lakanto)
- avocado oil for cooking
- few c of broccoli sprouts washed and dried
- 14 ounces / 4000g riced cauliflower, plus coconut aminos and wine vinegar +avocado oil

Preparation

1 In a large pan using low to medium heat, add some avocado oil. Stir in onions and stir regularly until onions are caramelized. Add one teaspoon of water at a time if necessary.

2 Mix the sauce ingredients: coconut aminos, cooking wine, Chinese five-spice, and monk fruit sweetener while the onions are cooking. Add the water to this mix before adding to the pan.

3 When the onions are caramelized, put them in a bowl, Add more avocado oil to the pan. Add the smashed garlic cloves. Infuse the oil with garlic for a couple of mins. Take the garlic out, chop it finely and add it to the onions bowl.

4 Increase heat to medium and begin cooking the pork belly slices in batches. When a batch is nicely browned, take it out and put it in the onion's bowl and add the next. Do this until you are finished with the pork belly. The pork belly will release a lot of fat, and I removed (with a spoon) most of it. Leave enough to cover the pan and coat all the ingredients. Add everything from the bowl back to the pan, mix well and add the sauce you prepared along with the water. Bring to a boil, cover and reduce heat. Simmer for half-hour to 40 mins until the sauce has thickened and reduced.

5 When the pork belly is almost ready, add some avocado oil to a different large pan, put in the cauliflower and sauté briefly. Drizzle coconut aminos and cooking wine over the cauliflower. Add salt if necessary. Cook the rice for a couple of mins until crunchy. Taste, adjust, and cook to your liking, but mushy is not nice.

6 Place the vegetable rice, pork belly, and broccoli sprouts in a serving bowl and garnish with sliced green onion.

Alaskan Salmon Cakes with Spinach Pesto and Avocado

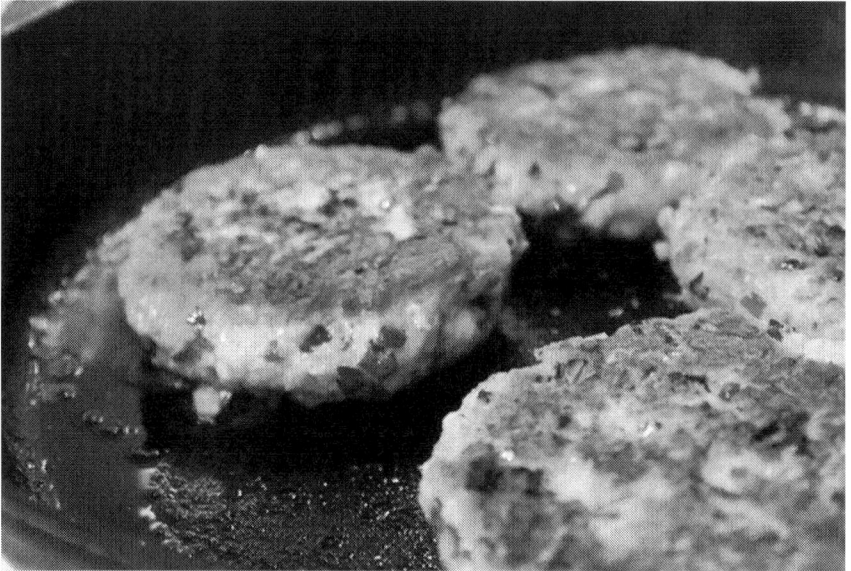

If you love salmon, then this is just the recipe you'll want to make and eat again and again. Salmon cakes are served over a spinach pesto and a thinly sliced avocado on the side. This is an easy, breezy delicious dinner idea!

Time Needed for Preparation: 30 Mins
Time Needed for Cooking: 30 Mins
Makes: 8-10

Salmon Cakes

- Twenty ounces raw Alaskan salmon, skins removed and finely chopped
- One-third c avocado mayonnaise - Primal Kitchen or homemade
- A handful of chopped celery – approximately one-half c
- A handful of chopped dill – approximately one-fourth c

- A handful of celeriac + carrots – approximately one-half c, mixed
- One-half red onion, chopped
- One and one-half to Two t. old bay seasoning
- One-half lemon, juice
- zest of one organic lemon
- ¾ t. salt
- Pepper
- 4-5 T. almond flour
- Optional: One-Two t. of Dijon mustard (You can use homemade mayonnaise which has a lot of mustard in it
- Optional: One-Two T. cassava flour, if you feel the mixture is too moist. This may depend on the thickness of your mayonnaise.
- More almond flour for coating (about ¾ c)
- Coconut or avocado oil for frying

Spinach Pesto

- One garlic clove
- 7-8 c of organic baby spinach
- One T. lemon juice
- A handful of pecans, walnuts, a mix of nuts or nuts of your choice
- One-fourth c grated aged, hard cheese like Parmigiano, Pecorino Romano, or Mancengo
- One-third c extra virgin olive oil – add more to get the desired consistency
- salt and pepper

Preparation

Salmon Cakes

1 Add the veggies In a food processor or blender and mix until finely chopped and well-mixed. Try not to over mix, but too-big pieces might not allow the cakes to hold together well.

2 Finely chop the salmon and mix it with the veggies, spices, mayonnaise, and flour. Make patties with your hands and coat them with almond flour. Place in the refrigerator before cooking for 1 to 2 hours.

3 Fry the salmon cakes on the stove in coconut or avocado oil, cooking on each side until golden brown. Handle carefully and not rough or they can break apart. So they don't stick to the pan, be sure there is enough oil.

Spinach Pesto

1 Add the spinach, nuts, cheese, and garlic to a food processor and mix until (almost) pureed. While the processor is on low speed, begin to add extra virgin olive oil. Adjust the consistency depending on your taste.

2 Add salt and pepper, and lemon juice.

3 Serve all with one-half sliced avocado, lemon wedges, and add some hot sauce if you like.

Salmon – a great seafood choice. It is rich in omega-3 fatty acids, high in essential B vitamins, a great source of protein, a good source of potassium, and loaded with selenium. It may benefit weight control and help reduce the risk of heart disease. Impressive!

Try to only eat salmon and other seafood that is freshly caught. The American Heart Association states that eating at least two servings of 3.5-ounce fatty fish like salmon every week is recommended. Wild Alaskan salmon is the healthiest salmon as it lives on a natural diet and the calorie and fat content are lower compared to a farmed salmon.

Wild Shrimp with Greens & Lemon Oil

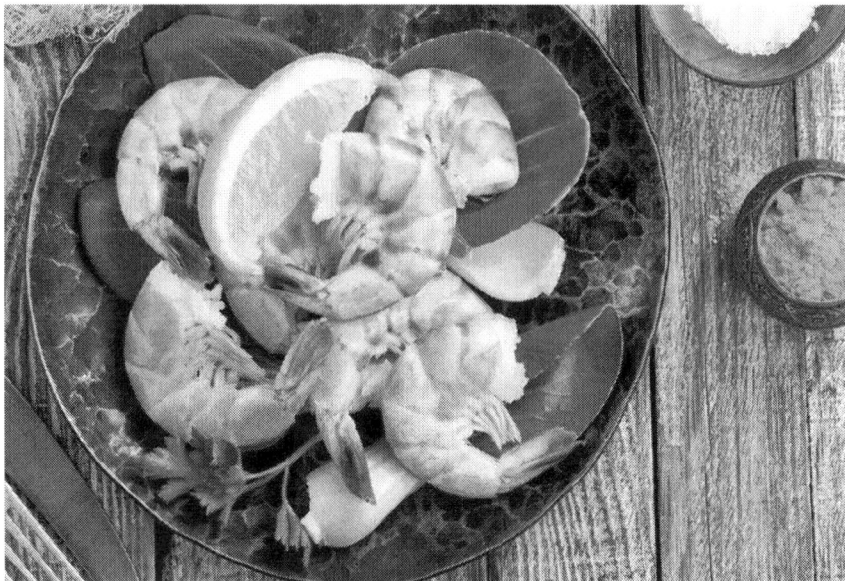

Time Needed for Preparation & Cooking: 15 Mins
Makes: 4

- One lb. wild-caught shelled jumbo shrimp
- Two sliced cloves garlic
- 4 strips lemon zest
- One-half c extra virgin olive oil (plus additional for brushing)
- sea salt
- One pinch red pepper
- One-half c chopped fresh parsley
- 5 ounces mixed greens
- white wine vinegar for sprinkling

Preparation

1 In a small pot, heat the oil, garlic, red pepper, lemon zest, and one-fourth teaspoon salt over medium heat. Cook until sizzling for two-three mins.

2   Take a large skillet and brush it with a small amount of olive oil. Preheat over medium heat.

3   Place the shrimp in the skillet. Cover the skillet and cook without moving them until opaque throughout or for three-five mins.

4   Place the shrimp, lemon oil, and parsley and toss to combine in a large bowl. Serve the greens on 4 plates, topping them off with the shrimp. Drizzle the remaining dressing at the bottom of the bowl over the greens. Sprinkle with white wine vinegar.

Chicken and Goat Cheese Enchiladas

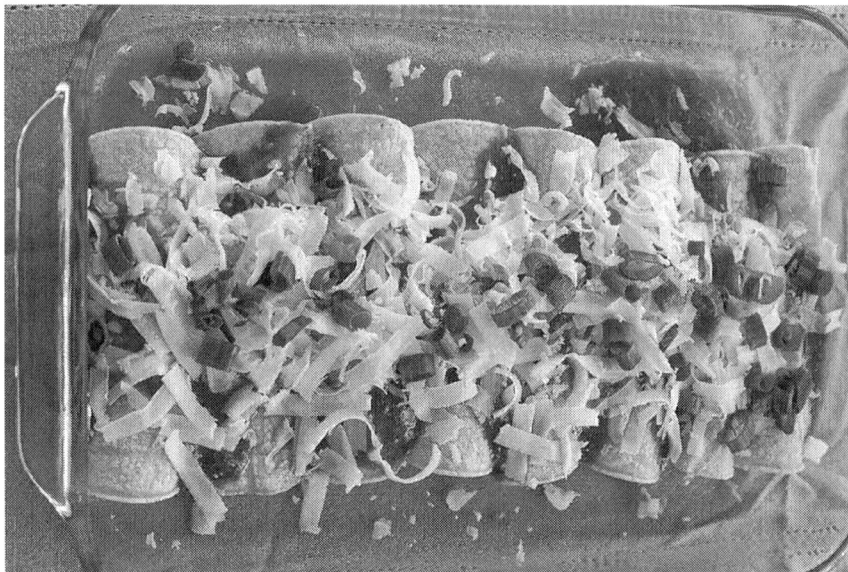

Here's a dish that you'll enjoy if you like enchiladas and have that craving for Mexican food!

Time Needed for Preparation: Thirty Mins
Overall Time Required: 45 Mins
Makes: 8 enchiladas

*Does not include time needed for cooking chicken and tortillas (if you don't have some already made)

Ingredients

- 8 ounces pastured chicken cooked and shredded
- Two T. olive oil
- Two c broth, divided
- One chopped white onion
- One-fourth t. paprika
- sea salt
- black pepper
- cloves garlic, peeled
- 8 ounces shiitake mushrooms – chopped

- 8 ounces goat cheese - crumbled
- One t. coconut aminos
- One-half t. dried oregano
- t. apple cider vinegar
- One teaspoon granular sweetener
- One-half t. ground cumin
- cassava flour tortillas – warmed*
- Fresh cilantro chopped and hot sauce for serving

*see Chapter Two on how to make 5-minute Cassava Flour Tortillas

Preparation

1 The olive oil should be heated In a large skillet, heat over medium-high heat. Mix in mushrooms and onions. Stir often about 6-8 mins until they soften.

2 Add the chicken, one-half c broth, one-fourth teaspoon pepper, and one-half teaspoon salt.

3 Heat should be reduced to medium. Stir often, until most of the liquid is absorbed or for about three-four mins. Transfer the chicken to a large bowl. Mix in half the goat cheese.

4 Make the adobo sauce by pulsing the remaining broth, cider vinegar, garlic, coconut aminos, two teaspoons sea salt, cumin, sweetener, oregano, and paprika in a blender until very, very smooth or for about three mins.

5 Using 9 x 13-inch glass baking dish, pour one-half c of the adobo sauce into the bottom of the dish. Using a one-fourth-c as a scoop, roll up the mushroom mixture into each tortilla side, pour the remaining adobo sauce evenly on top and sprinkle the remainder of the goat cheese. Bake in the oven at three hundred fifty degrees Fahrenheit. The sauce should be bubbling and the goat cheese should be melted in about 15 mins.

6   Sprinkle with cilantro and hot sauce.

Why goat cheese? A goat's milk rather than a cow's is a bit lower in fat than the cheese from cow's milk. It also provides a slightly tangy taste that livens up any dish. It can make practically anything taste better.

Lectin-Free Chili

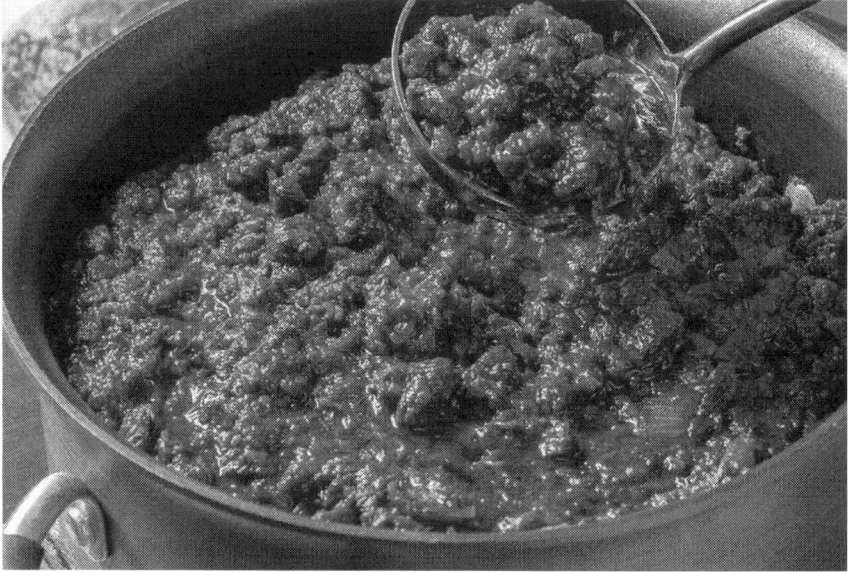

We can't have a cookbook without a good bowl of chili and some salads that are super easy to make.

Time Needed for Preparation: Fifteen mins
Overall Time required: Six hours and fifteen mins
Makes: 8

- Two pounds ground beef (grass-fed)
- 4 minced cloves of garlic
- One finely diced medium onion
- One t. avocado oil, divided
- Three finely diced celery ribs
- sea salt
- black pepper
- Two T. chili powder
- One-fourth t. ground cinnamon
- Two t. ground cumin
- pinch ground cloves
- One 15-ounces can sweet potato purée

- Three ounces pine nuts
- One T. sauce from preserved chipotles in adobo
- Two t. red wine vinegar
- Two c grass-fed beef broth
- Two t. coconut aminos
- sour cream, for serving (optional)
- For garnish slice lime wedges and scallions

Preparation

1   Add one pound ground beef and one-half t. salt to a large skillet over high heat with one tsp oil. Brown and break the meat apart. Put the meat into a slow-cooker and repeat with the one lb. of beef that remains.

2   Lower the heat to medium. Heat up the remaining oil. Mix the garlic, celery and onion. Cook for 5 mins until soft.

3   Mix in the chili powder, cumin, cloves, and cinnamon, cooking for one minute while stirring. Pour in the broth, scraping the bottom of the pan so all the mixture is transferred to the pot.

4   Mix the sweet potato puree, adobo sauce, wine vinegar, pine nuts, coconut aminos, salt, and pepper. Cover the slow cooker and cook for 6 hours. Serve with, lime wedges, scallions, and sour cream, if desired.

All the products for this and many of the recipes in this book can be purchased on Amazon.com and Thrive Market https://www.thrivemarket.com/

Steak & Spinach Salad

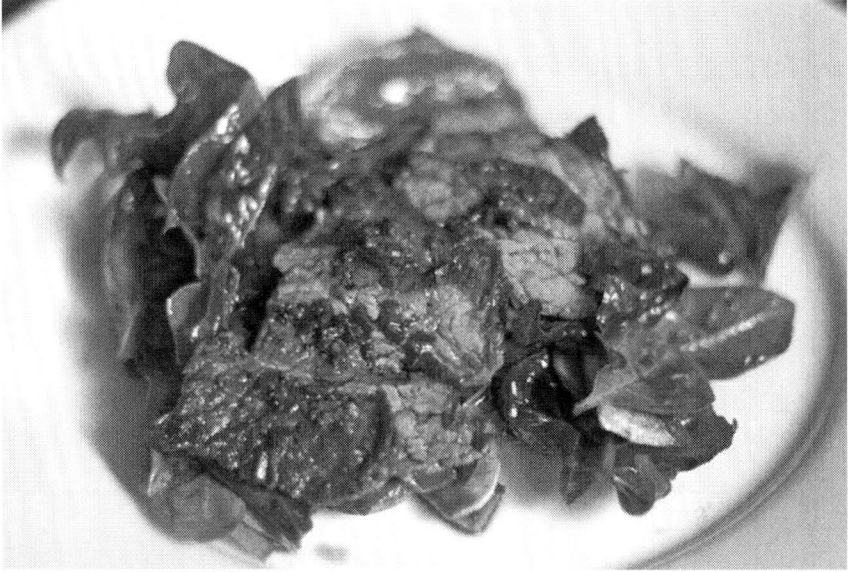

Time Needed for Preparation and Cooking: Thirty Mins
Makes: 2-4

- One lb. sliced and cooked grass-fed steak
- One c shirataki rice (drained & rinsed)
- 5 ounces baby spinach
- Two T. toasted pine nuts

Yogurt Dressing

Combine:

- Two teaspoons thyme leaves
- Two tablespoons wine vinegar (red)
- One c whole goat/sheep milk yogurt
- salt & pepper

Preparation

1   Cook the steak 4 mins each side for medium-rare and longer for well-done.

2   Whisk all the ingredients for yogurt dressing until totally blended.

Salmon & Orange Salad w. Dijon Vinaigrette

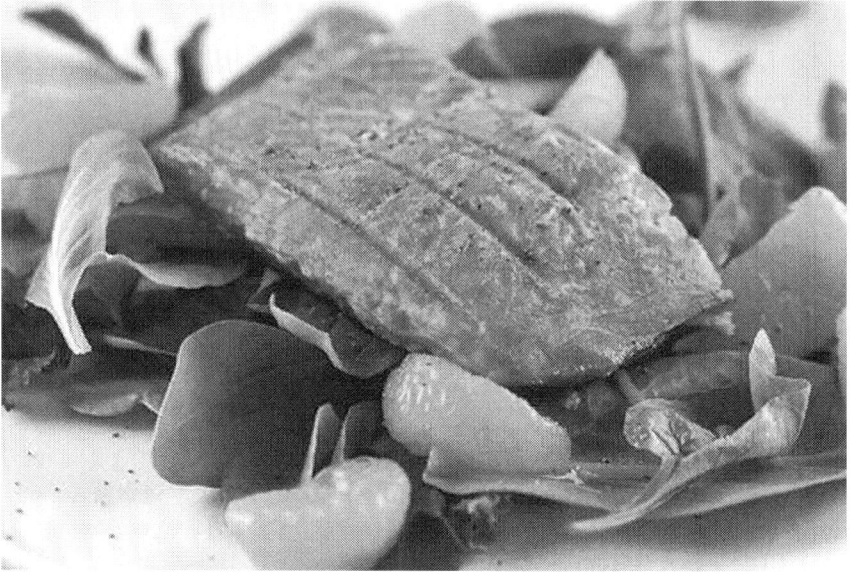

Time Needed for Preparation: Fifteen Mins
Makes: 2-4

Toss together:

- One lb. broiled or canned wild salmon - flaked
- 8 ounces baby spinach
- peeled and sectioned Navel oranges
- One small thinly sliced red onion
- 8 ounces real Feta cheese, crumbled
- One-third c toasted hazelnuts – chopped

Dijon Vinaigrette

- One t. Dijon mustard
- One T. chopped fresh dill
- Three T. white wine vinegar
- 4 T. olive oil - extra virgin
- Juice of One lemon
- Salt to taste

Preparation:

1   Toss all the ingredients for salad together in a large salad bowl.

2   Mix and whisk the ingredients for the Dijon vinaigrette.

3   Pour over the salad.

As you begin to learn to cook and eat differently, there is the grieving process that goes along with a lectin-free diet. There will be times when you really want to eat your old comfort foods like pasta or rice. The urges will be strong at times and you may not even want to go out to eat for fear you'll be too tempted and the frustration of trying to decide what you can eat will be just too much of a hassle.

Let's look at this in another way. You are taking care of your health and body, the only one you're going to have in this life. Persevere and do whatever it takes to avoid temptation and the foods that, quite frankly, don't do your health any good, not to mention block your efforts to lose weight.

There are ways of replacing the old with new and better. You may even be able to convert some of your longed-for dishes into lectin-free meals.

Chapter Five: Lectin-Free Dessert Recipes

Almost everyone loves dessert! There are those who suggest that life is short and unpredictable so eat dessert first. This chapter may just convince some of you to do just that!

First up is what some wouldn't think of as a dessert, but if you love chocolate in any form, this classic hot chocolate recipe is just the thing for a winter's night and makes for an unbelievable dessert.

Classic Hot Chocolate

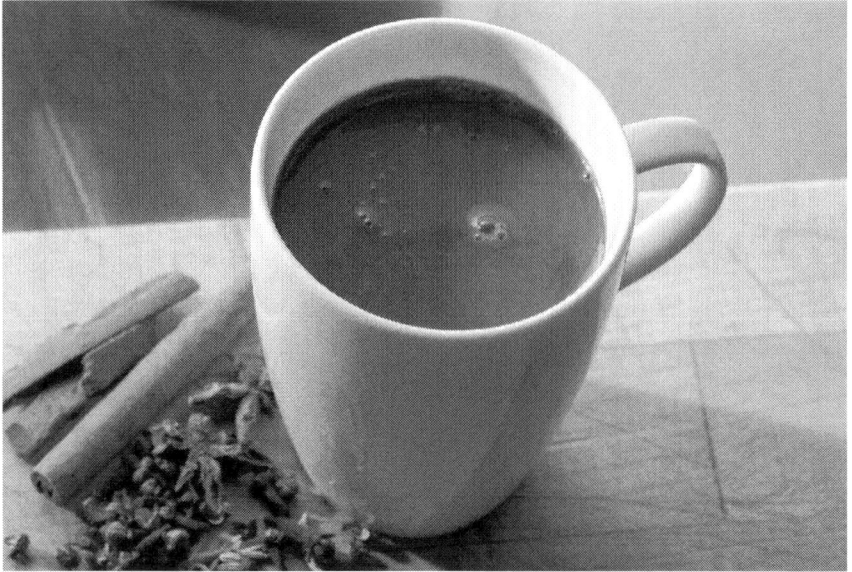

Time Needed for Preparation: Ten Mins
Makes: Two

- Three c light Coconut Milk*
- One-fourth c (Twenty g) Dutch-processed cocoa powder
- One-half t. liquid Stevia
- One t. vanilla extract
- One t. virgin Coconut Oil
- One-fourth t. salt – always use a bit of salt when using stevia

Preparation

1 Use a personal-sized blender or mini food processor and combine one cup of coconut milk with all of the cocoa powder, coconut oil, vanilla extract, stevia, and salt. Blend until smooth.

2   Pour into a medium sauce pot. Cook over high heat. Add in the remaining coconut milk. Reduce the heat and simmer the mixture to a light boil.

3   Pour into two cups and savor!

Dark chocolate can positively affect your health. Full of nutrients, dark chocolate comes from the seed of the cocoa tree and is one of the best sources of antioxidants. Research has shown that dark chocolate (not chocolate loaded with sugar) can lower the risk of heart disease and improve your health. (Gunnars, 2018)(Cross, Poppy, 2014)

3.5 ounces (10-grams) of dark chocolate containing 70-85% cocoa has 11 grams of fiber and the recommended daily intake (RDI) of the following: 58% of magnesium, 67% iron, 98% manganese, and 89% copper. It also contains a good amount of zinc, selenium, potassium, and phosphorus.

Rich Dark Chocolate Brownies with Large Sea Salt Flakes

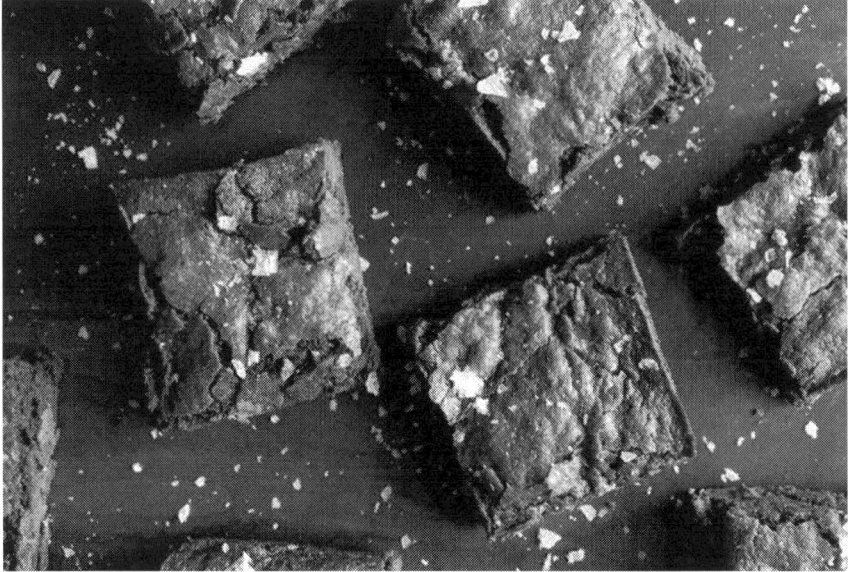

The sweet and the salty all rolled into these unbelievable lectin-free brownies. Perfect with your hot chocolate or all by themselves. It has the perfect balance of softness, airiness, chewiness, and richness. Totally decadent!

Time Needed for Preparation and Cooking: One Hr. Fifteen Mins Makes: 8 large squares

Ganache

- One-half c (112 grams) melted vegan butter or coconut oil
- 12 grams (12 T.) of Dutch-processed cocoa powder
- 8 ounces dark chocolate chips or chopped dark chocolate

Wet Ingredients

- 4 T. Vegan Egg powder – Follow Your Heart brand

- One t. vanilla extract
- One-half c +Two tablespoons (5 ounces) ice cold water
- One t. salt
- One c (One9Two grams) erythritol or granular Swerve

Dry Ingredients

- One-half c (34 grams) sorghum flour
- One-half c (32grams) cassava flour
- One-fourth c (24 grams) Dutch-processed cocoa powder
- One-fourth t. xanthan gum

Topping – totally optional

- Large sea salt flakes

Preparation

1 Cut a piece of parchment paper to fit a 9.25 x 4.25-inches loaf pan.

2 Use the excess paper on each side. This will help you remove the brownies from the pan later on. If your pan has a problem with sticking, coat with a light layer of coconut oil.

3 Pre-heat oven to Three hundred fifty degrees Fahrenheit.

4 Whisk the water and Vegan Egg powder together in either a stand-up mixer bowl using a whisk attachment or in a large bowl with an electric hand whisk. Make sure the mixture is thoroughly combined for approximately two mins.

5 Make the ganache by placing chocolate chips and cocoa powder in a small bowl. Melt buttery coconut

81

oil in a small pot until it's hot to the touch or for about 175 degrees Fahrenheit.

6 Pour the melted oil over chocolate chips & cocoa powder. Allow it to sit for 5 mins, untouched. After 5 mins, stir it until all of the chocolate has melted and the mixture is smooth.

7 Once the egg mixture is light and fluffy, reduce the speed to low and slowly pour in chocolate ganache. If mixing by hand, make sure to mix until chocolate is fully incorporated.

8 Remove bowl from mixer. Sift in all of the dry ingredients on top of the chocolate egg mixture. Gently fold with a spatula until dry ingredients are no longer visible.

9 Transfer the batter to the prepped loaf pan and spread out with a spatula. Make sure the top is smooth and flat. Bake in the oven for twenty mins.

10 Remove the loaf pan from oven. Bang the bottom of the pan on the counter three times. This creates flat brownies instead of brownies with an indented center.

11 Sprinkle on a few heavy pinches of large sea salt flakes. Place the pan back into the oven for another twenty mins.

12 Place pan on cooling rack for ten mins then transfer the brownies directly to the rack using the parchment sling.

13 Let it cool for at least 15 more mins before cutting. They'll be very fudgy if you eat them while they're warm. For a cleaner cut and well-rounded brownies, allow them to cool for an hour.

14 Use a sharp chef's knife to cut them. Cut once down the middle vertically and three times across horizontally, thus creating 8 square pieces.

15 The brownies can be stored at room temperature up to three days. If you want to warm up the brownies, re-heat for about 6 mins in the oven at three hundred fifty degrees Fahrenheit oven until warm.

16 Enjoy!

Chocolate and Raspberry Ice Cream Squares

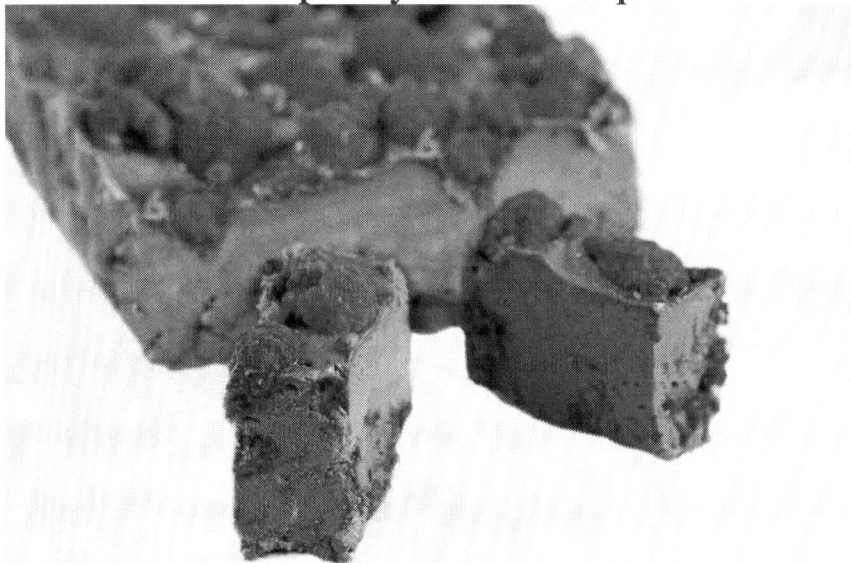

This dessert can actually be prepared in five mins. Chocolate and raspberry ice cream squares is an easy a dessert and totally delicious. Raspberries are an excellent source of vitamin C, high in antioxidants, and a good source of dietary fiber.

Time Needed for Preparation: 5 Mins
Inactive: Two Hours
Makes: Ten - Twelve small squares

Ice Cream

- One can organic full-fat coconut milk (13.5 ounces can)
- One-fourth c date nectar – organic
- Two organic (pitted) avocados
- One-half c cacao powder - raw
- One-fourth t. Himalayan pink salt
- One-fourth t. organic vanilla bean powder

Add

- One c organic raspberries, freeze-dried

Topping

- One-half c organic raspberries, freeze-dried

Preparation

1 ***Pre-preparation*** – Freeze the 13.5 ounces can of full-fat coconut milk for one hour before beginning the recipe. The fat of the coconut milk is what you'll be using, not the water. If you want to make this dessert frequently, always keep a can in the refrigerator to use when you want it.

2 Take out the coconut milk from the freezer. Use only the hardened "fat" portion of the can and add to a mixer or blender. A smoothie can be made from the remaining coconut water.

3 Into the mixer or blender, mix all the ingredients for the ice cream and blend until smooth and creamy.

4 Mix in one c of freeze-dried raspberries and stir by hand. Do not use a mixer or blender.

5 In an 8 x 5 bread pan lined with parchment paper, take the entire mixture and spread evenly in the pan.

6 Take one-half of freeze-dried raspberries as the topping and spread evenly across the top. Let the mixture harden in the pan by putting it in the freezer for about two-three hours.

7 Cut the hardened ice cream into rectangular bar pieces or small square pieces.

8   In order to preserve the ice cream, store in an air-tight
    BPA-free container. Do not leave the remainder of the ice
    cream out at room temperature, otherwise, they will
    soften.

9   Indulge and enjoy!

Sugar-Free White Chocolate

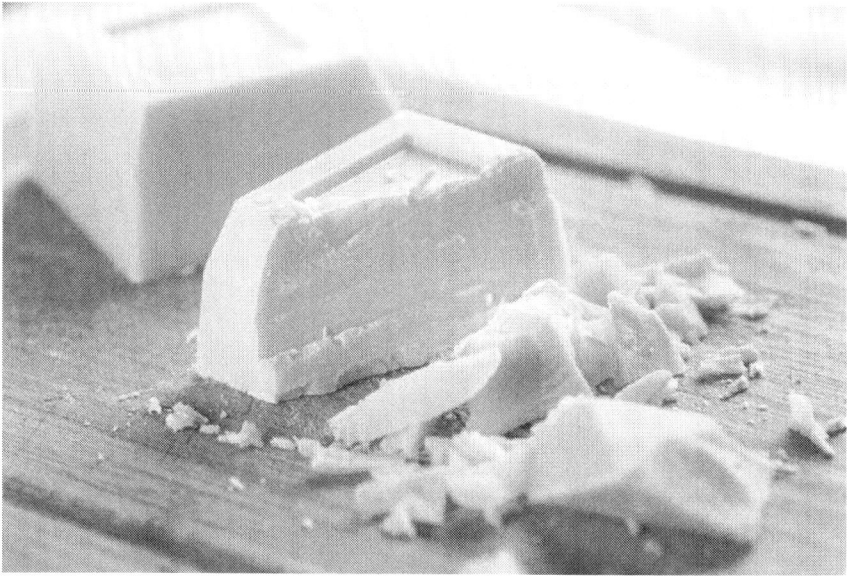

Another chocolate dessert treats, but this time it is white chocolate, just as scrumptious as all the other chocolate desserts.

Time Needed for Preparation: Thirty Mins
Inactive: One-Two Hours
Makes: 6-8 Squares

- 4 ounces. Cocoa Butter
- One large egg yolk (beaten with a fork)
- One T. Coconut Oil
- One-fourth c Coconut Milk Powder
- One-fourth c Powdered erythritol (Swerve Confection)
- One-half t. Vanilla extract
- 1/16 t. Sea Salt

Preparation

1   Break the cocoa butter discs into small pieces.

2 Place the cocoa butter, beaten egg yolk, and coconut oil into top container of double boiler. Add water to the bottom part of the boiler and place it on low heat. Slowly melt the cocoa butter. Don't allow it to get too hot. Once the mixture melts, remove from heat.

3 Mix in the sweetener and stir letting it dissolve completely. Stir in the coconut milk powder, the vanilla extract, and sea salt.

4 Pour into a pan lined with parchment paper. Refrigerate until hardened.

5 Cut into various sized squares once hard.

6 Enjoy!

Snickerdoodle Cookies

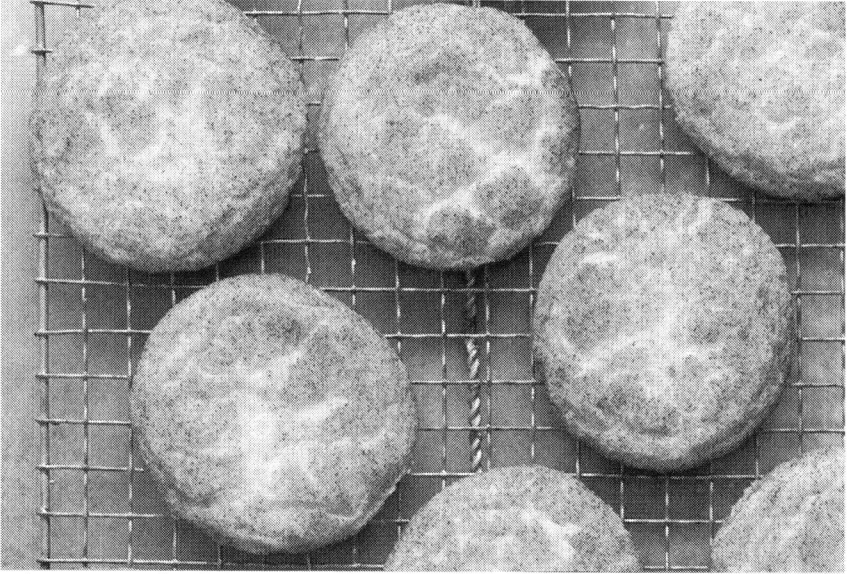

Time Needed for Preparation: Ten mins
Time Needed for Cooking: Twelve Mins
Makes: 18 small cookies

- One egg
- One-fourth c softened butter
- Two c almond flour
- 4 T. Lakanto Golden
- One t. vanilla
- pinch salt

Cinnamon Sugar mix

- Two T. Lakanto Golden
- One t. cinnamon

Preparation

1   Heat oven to three hundred fifty degrees Fahrenheit.

2   Blend together the Lakanto Golden and butter.

3   Add the almond, flour, vanilla, egg, and salt. Mix together
    until well incorporated.

4   Portion the mixture into small balls of dough. For ease,
    measure out the dough using a spoon but you can also use
    a small ice cream scoop. Try to keep the cookies small.
    There will be more of them to enjoy!

5   In a shallow bowl, mix together Lakanto golden and
    cinnamon. Roll each ball of dough over the mixture. Put
    into the baking tray.

6   Bake until the bottoms of the cookies are just beginning
    to brown, about twelve-thirteen mins.

7   Cool on cooling rack and enjoy.

Almond Flour Sugar-Free Chocolate Cookies

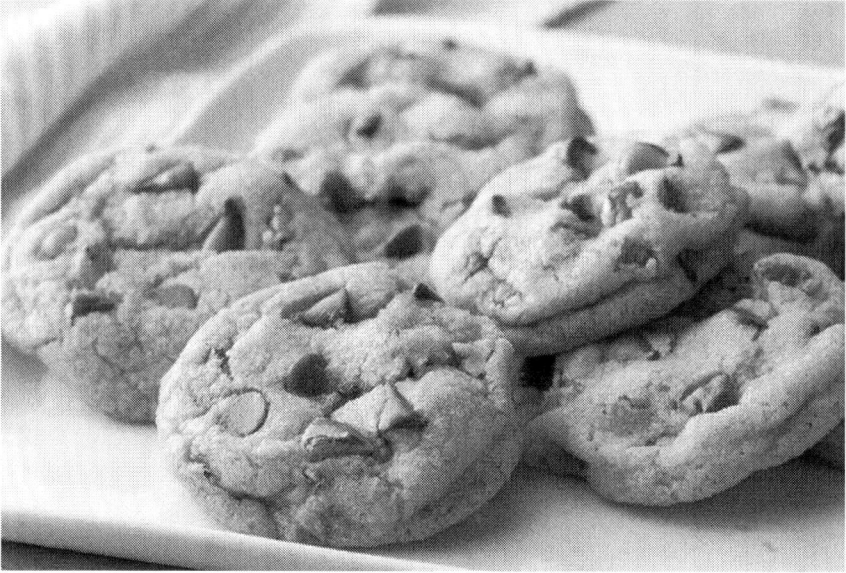

Time Needed for Preparation: Thirty Mins
Time Needed for Cooking: 8-9 Mins
Makes: 32 cookies

- T. maple flavored syrup (suggest Lakanto brand)
- T. solid coconut oil
- Two large eggs – pastured raised
- c almond flour
- One t. baking soda
- One-half t. sea salt – fine grain
- Two t. vanilla extract
- One c dark chocolate chips (add more for topping if desired)

Preparation

1 Line a baking sheet with parchment paper. Heat oven to Three 75 degrees F

2   Mix the Lakanto Maple Syrup and the coconut oil in a large bowl. Whisk until blended. Add egg and vanilla extract. Whisk quickly until completely blended.

3   Using another bowl, combine the salt, baking soda and almond flour. Combine flour mixture to the wet ingredients. Blend and add chocolate chips.

4   Scoop out the dough with an ice cream scoop, medium in size. Place scoops on the baking sheet approximately two inches apart. Press each cookie down gently, but do not flatten.

5   Bake the cookies for about 8-9 mins until they are set and lightly browned around the edges. Take the baking sheet out of the oven and allow the cookies to cool for 5 mins. Move the cookies to a wire rack to cool.

Orange Cranberry Muffins

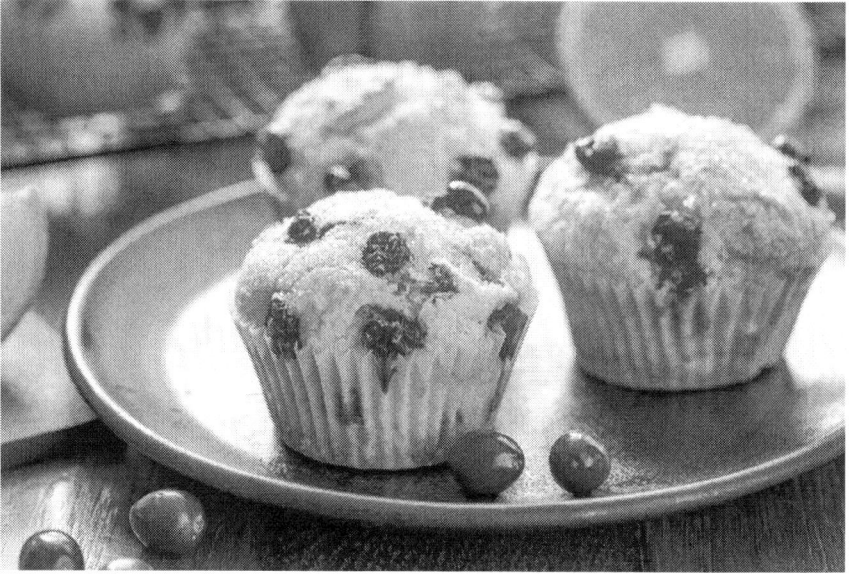

Time Needed for Preparation: Twenty Mins
Time Needed for Cooking: 30 Mins
Makes: 12 Muffins

- One c organic fresh cranberries
- One One-half c blanched almond flour – packed
- One-fourth c coconut flour – packed
- One t. baking soda
- Three eggs – pasture raised
- T. orange juice
- One-half t. salt
- One t. vanilla extract
- Three T. Monkfruit sweetener or Swerve
- One-fourth c full-fat coconut milk (in a can)
- One-Two T. poppy seeds
- One-fourth c avocado oil
- One T. lemon juice
- Zest of Three organic oranges
- Zest of One organic lemon

Preparation

1 Heat the oven to three hundred fifty degrees Fahrenheit. Fill a muffin cup with 12 paper muffin cups. Wash and dry the cranberries.

2 Mix the coconut flour, baking soda, almond flour, salt bowl. In a second bowl, add the eggs, avocado oil, coconut milk, vanilla, orange and lemon zest, the orange and lemon juices, and the monk fruit.

3 Mix the wet and the dry ingredients until thoroughly combined. Gently mix in the cranberries to the dough with a spatula.

4 Begin adding dough into the muffin cup using a large spoon. Sprinkle some poppy seeds across the top.

5 Bake for 25-30 mins. Don't over-bake the cupcakes. Monitor the oven to prevent this.

*The flour measurement refers to "packed." The cup should be packed. Press down with the back of a spoon or your hand until you reach the one cup (or one-fourth cup) mark. Coconut and almond flours can be fluffy, so if you don't add the correct amount, your cake will end up being too moist and can fall apart.

Mint Chocolate Cookies

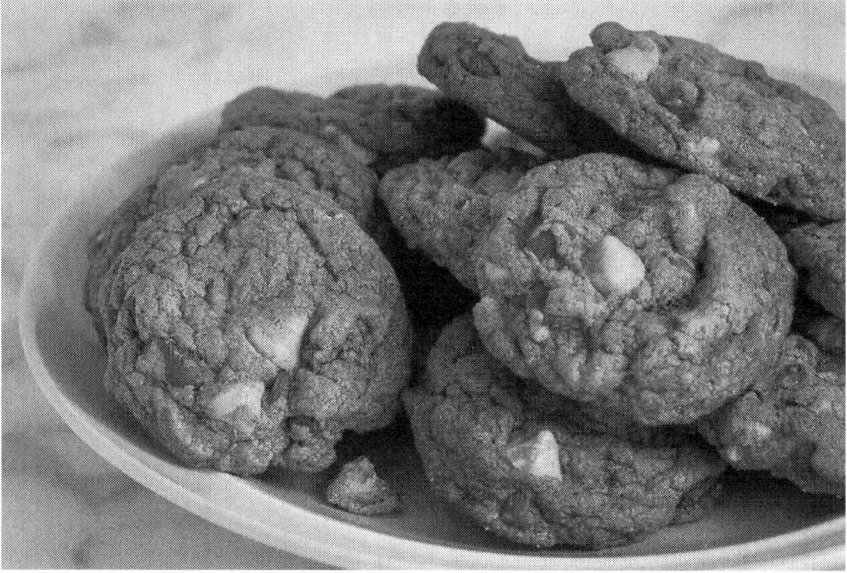

Time Needed for Preparation: Thirty Mins
Time Needed for Cooking: Ten-twelve Mins
Makes: 12 Cookies

- One c almond butter - creamy
- Two/Three c confectioner's Swerve (erythritol)
- Two T. blanched almond meal
- Two T. non-Dutched cocoa powder
- One T. coconut flour
- Two T. of water
- One t. baking soda
- Two large omega-Three or pastured eggs or Vegan Eggs
- Two T. melted salted butter or coconut oil
- One and one-half t. pure peppermint extract
- One-fourth c chopped bittersweet chocolate

Preparation

1   Using a baking sheet, line with parchment paper.

2   Heat oven to three hundred fifty degrees Fahrenheit.

3   Mix the cocoa powder, almond butter, erythritol, almond meal, coconut flour, water, eggs, butter or oil, baking soda, and peppermint extract in a mixing bowl.

4   Use a stand mixer or whisk in manually combining all the ingredients.

5   Fold in the chocolate. Form cookie dough into two-inch balls to make 12 cookies or somewhat smaller to make 18 cookies.

6   On the prepared baking sheet, place the cookie dough balls allowing them enough room to spread while baking.

7   The cookies will bake within ten to twelve mins. Take out of the oven. Let the cookies cool prior to eating. Store the extra cookies up to three to four days in an airtight container.

We all love snacks, and while we're dieting, we tend to get anxious about what we can eat as a snack. This chapter will give you a number of great ideas that will help you with your snacking dilemma. All are lectin-free and low calorie. No worries!

Sweet Potato Toast

An excellent snack for those of us who have a limited amount of time to eat breakfast or have to have sweet potato craving!

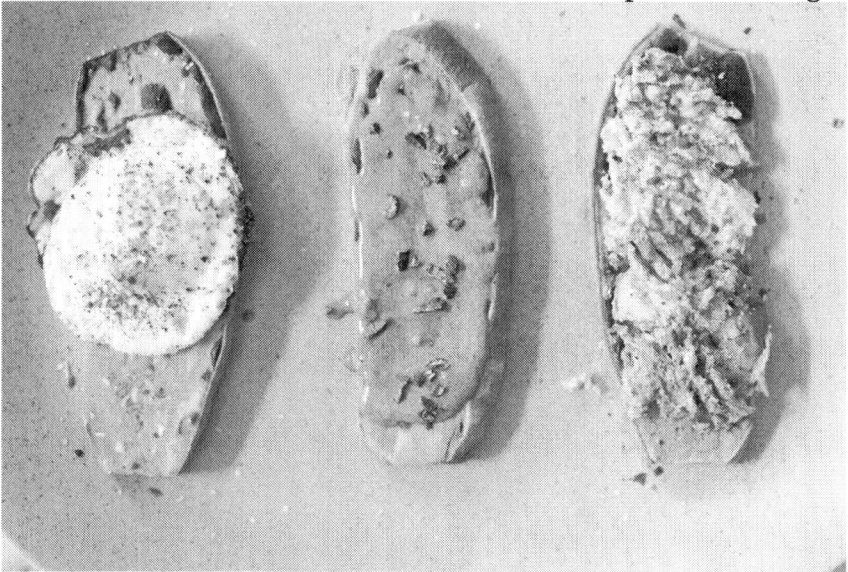

Time Needed for Preparation: Ten mins
Time Needed for Cooking: Fifteen-twenty mins

Preparation

1   Slice a sweet potato very thin length-wise into one-fourth-inch slices. Use organic sweet potatoes because you'll be eating the skin. You may want to cut off the ends of the ends to make the potato more stable when slicing.

2   In a toaster oven or regular oven, cook the slices at four hundred fifty degrees Fahrenheit for 15-25 mins, flipping once until they are tender and brown in spots.

3   Remove and enjoy them immediately with your favorite toppings or allow them to cool and freeze them up to three months. When you're ready to use them, just pop them in the toaster oven or regular oven and reheat them.

Some topping ideas

- Avocado and sliced hard-boiled eggs
- Avocado
- Butter and Sea Salt
- Scrambled eggs – Omega Three or VeganEgg
- Avocado, egg, goat cheese
- Spinach and goat cheese
- Lox and goat cheese

There are quite a number of toppings that you can put on these sweet potato toasts and make them a snack treat. They're great for after-school snacks for the kids or a midday pick-me-up.

Classic Guacamole

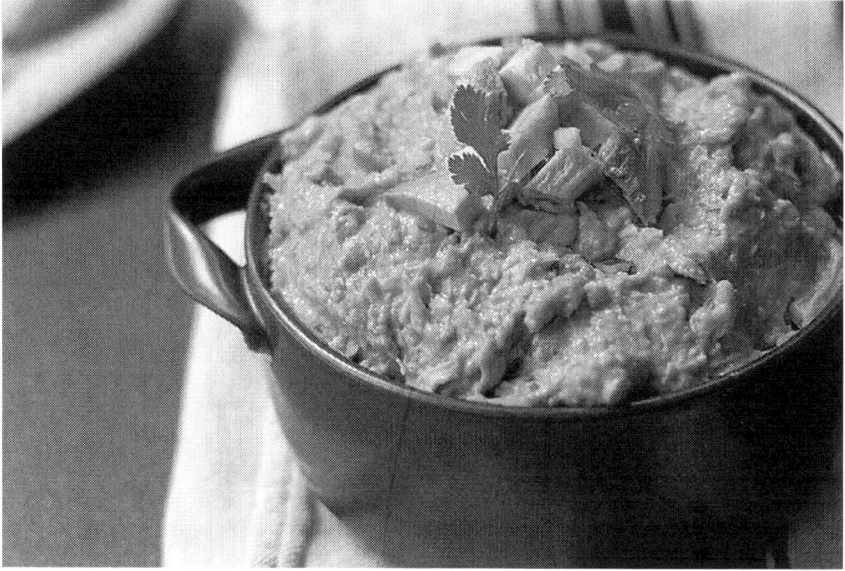

One healthy dip that's are lectin-free and can be a snack dip for almost everything!

Time Needed for Preparation: 5 Mins

- Two cut and smashed ripe avocados
- Juice of One lime
- Two tbsp fresh chopped cilantro
- Dash of chalula
- Salt
- Pepper

Preparation

1   Mash with a fork combine avocados, cilantro, lime juice, salt, and pepper.

2   Top with chalula.

3   Grab a chip, carrot, or celery stick. Spread it on a sweet potato toast.

Artichoke Pesto

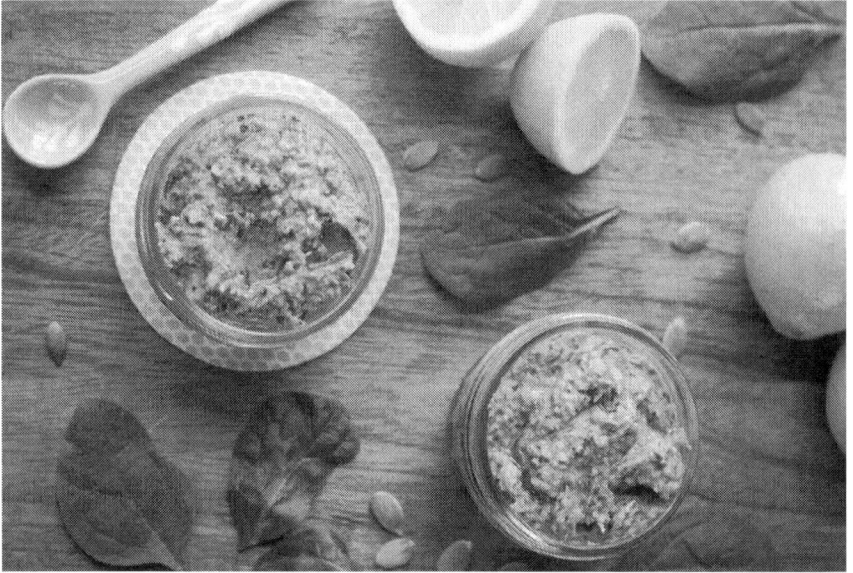

Time Needed for Preparation: Ten Mins

- One-half c sheep or goats milk ricotta
- One-half c fresh basil leaves
- One-half c chopped artichoke hearts
- One-fourth c olive oil
- One-fourth c pecorino romano, grated
- Salt
- Pepper

Preparation

1   Combine artichokes, basil, ricotta, olive oil, pecorino, salt, and pepper in processor. Blend until mixture has a smooth consistency.

2   Serve with celery sticks or sweet potato chips.

Sweet Hummus with Roasted Garlic

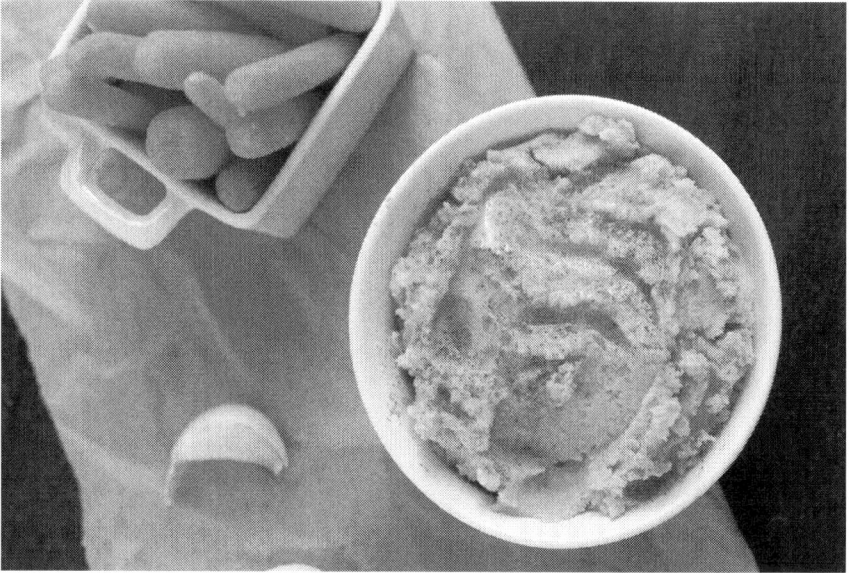

Time Needed for Preparation: Ten mins
Time Needed for Cooking: 35-40 Mins
Makes: 4-6

- One sweet potato, large, whole, washed and dried
- One t. ghee/avocado oil
- One heaping T. tahini
- 4-6 whole garlic cloves, unpeeled
- One-half lime – squeeze for juice
- few t. extra virgin olive oil
- sea salt
- raw vegetable sticks (for serving) – celery, carrots, cauliflower florets

Preparation

1   Heat oven to three hundred seventy-five degrees Fahrenheit.

2   Using a fork, poke holes in the sweet potato. Grease potato and garlic cloves with ghee/avocado oil and add them to a sheet pan.

3   Bake the garlic for about twenty-five mins and the potato for thirty to forty mins, depending on how large and dense your potato is. Allow the potato to cool down, peel the garlic.

4   When the potato is cool, peel it and add the flesh to a food processor. Add 2-4 garlic cloves (depending on how much you like garlic). Add lime juice, tahini, and some salt and process until smooth.

5   Adjust seasoning to your taste. You can add a few t. extra virgin olive oil to the mix or just add the oil on top of serving bowls (or both).

6   Serve with raw vegetable sticks or compliant crackers.

7   Place in an airtight container and refrigerate.

Rainbow Vegetables Oven Fries

- purple carrots, peeled, halved, and quartered lengthwise
- Peel and cut two medium sweet potatoes into one-fourth inch thick strips
- Peel and cut two medium yuca roots into one-fourth inch thick strips
- Two t. granulated garlic
- Three T. olive oil – extra virgin
- Two t. sea salt
- black pepper
- ¾ c full-fat sour cream
- Three tablespoons grainy mustard

Preparation

1   Heat oven to four hundred fifty degrees F. Place two baking sheets on top and bottom thirds of the oven.

2   Toss the carrots, sweet potatoes, yucca, olive oil, granulated garlic, salt, and several grinds of black pepper. Divide between the preheated baking sheets.

3   Total bake time is twenty mins until crisp and golden. Rotate the sheets between top and bottom, tossing the fries halfway.

4   Mix mustard, sour cream, and a generous grinding of pepper in a small bowl.

5   Serve fries on a serving platter with sweet hummus with roasted garlic dip or mustard dip.

Dark Chocolate Candy Crunch

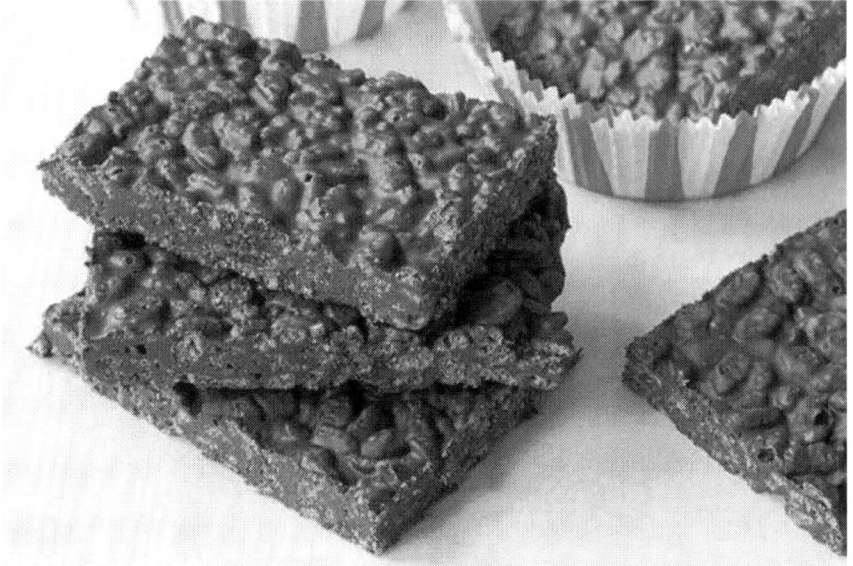

Crispy, crunchy lectin-free dark chocolate candy bars with added protein.

Time Needed for Preparation: Fifteen mins
Overall Time Required: 45 Mins
Makes: 24 Bars of Chocolate

- 24 ounces dark chocolate (72% or higher) pieces
- One-fourth c sesame seeds
- One-fourth c hemp hearts
- 1.5 c puffed millet
- Himalayan sea salt

Preparation

1 Completely melt the chocolate using a double boiler over simmering water. Let it cool slightly. In a small bowl, mix the seeds together and set aside two tablespoons to use as a topping.

2   Mix puffed millet and seeds into the melted chocolate.
    Scrape into a parchment lined 9×13 glass pan. Use a
    spatula to smooth out. Bang on the counter a few times to
    settle the contents. Sprinkle the reserved seeds over the
    top and generously grind sea salt over top.

3   Refrigerate for twenty-thirty mins. Remove from the
    fridge. Use a sharp knife to cut into approximately 24
    dark chocolate bars. Store in an airtight container– on the
    countertop in cool weather or in the refrigerator if it's
    summertime or a warm climate area.

Nuts as a Snack

Walnuts

One of the best foods to fight inflammation is walnuts. There was a time where we ate equal amounts of omega-6 fatty inflammatory acids and omega-3 anti-inflammatory acids. This balance aided the body to turn the inflammation off and on when needed.

Now, we eat an average of approximately twenty times more inflammatory fatty acids and the imbalance remains unchecked and can remain and linger. What your body needs is an increase in omega-3 fatty acid intake. They maintain intestinal wall integrity and reduce gut inflammation.

Walnuts are full of omega-3 fatty acid, antioxidants, and nutrients. A one-fourth cup of walnuts fiber, carbohydrates, protein, and 18 grams of fat. Walnuts are antioxidant polyphenols and have the highest amount of omega-3s that provides quite a wallop against chronic inflammation over other nuts.

It is a quick and snack that helps fight inflammation, support gut health, and quite a lot more.

Macadamia Nuts

Macadamia nuts are high in the "good" fat of monounsaturated fatty acid. They have been known to help reduce cholesterol levels. They are indigenous to Australia and named after John Macadam, a Scottish born chemist and physician. He promoted the cultivation of nuts in Australia.

They were introduced into Hawaii in 1881 and were used as an ornament. The first commercial orchards of macadamias were not planted until 1921 in Hawaii.

National Macadamia Nut Day is September 4th (mark your calendar!).

Macadamias are harvested when they fall fully ripened from the tree; they are not picked.

The macadamia shell is the hardest of all nut shells.

Pine Nuts

Pine nuts contain pinolenic acid. This activates the release of an appetite-suppressing hormone and may help with losing weight. They're also an excellent source of magnesium. This may help in fighting disease and boost energy.

Two-Minute Vanilla Mug Cake

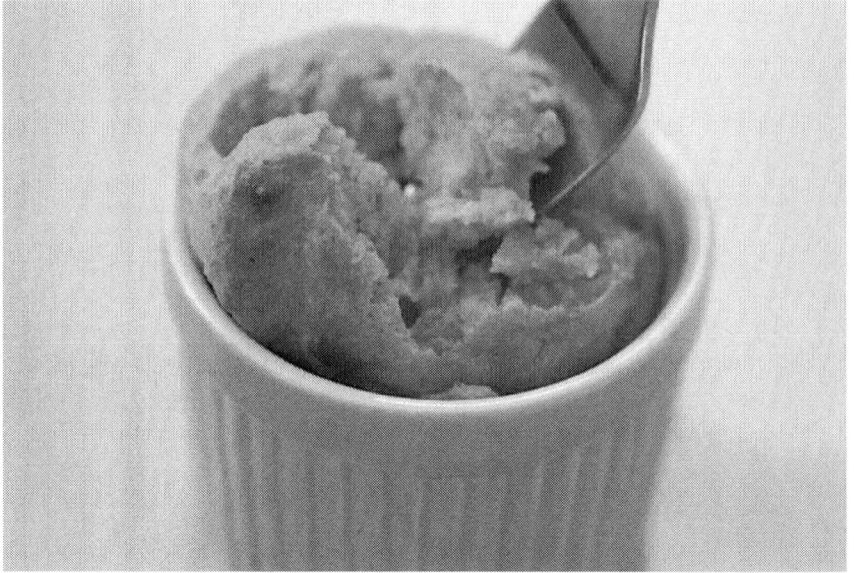

It is a fluffy, grain-free, and lectin-free vanilla muffin in a mug.

Time Needed for Preparation: Two mins
Time Needed for Cooking: One minute
Makes: One

- One large pastured or omega-3 egg beaten
- Two T. extra-virgin olive oil
- One T. coconut flour
- One T. tigernut flour
- One-half t. baking powder
- One-half t. vanilla
- Two teaspoons granular monk fruit sweetener
- One pinch sea salt
- One tablespoon seasonal fruit or dark chocolate chips (optional)

Preparation:

1   Combine the oil, egg, coconut flour, tigernut flour, baking powder, sweetener, vanilla, and salt into a mug that is microwave safe. Beat the mixture with a fork until the batter is smooth. Scrape the sides and bottom of the mug. Gently fold in the fruit or chocolate chips, whatever you desire.

2   Microwave for one minute and thirty seconds. Allow to cool for a minute. Once cool, scrape around the edges with a butter knife and shake the muffin onto a plate.

3   Serve topped with butter, seasonal fruit, or as is.

Tips and Tricks

When we begin a diet, we tend to stay on the straight and narrow for the first couple of weeks. In some cases, even the first 30 days. And then, we slip a little. We catch ourselves and climb back on that "diet wagon." And then we slip a little again, except it's a bigger slip than the first time. We get frustrated and hard on ourselves. Why did we do that? We're trying to lose weight here. But for some reason, we end up sabotaging the very plan that we try to set for ourselves.

Here are some tips and tricks that can help. It is, however, totally up to an individual to do what they can to follow and maintain their diet.

Lectin-free can be called a diet, but it is a matter of totally changing the way you look at all foods, not just the naughty ones like ice cream, cakes, or too many fries. It is the realization that lectins are not good for your gut, can cause diseases that you don't want, or can exacerbate diseases that may already exist within you.

If you have cravings, especially for say potato chips or some other type of chip we enjoyed in the past, there is the Sweet Potato Toast that you can make up in no time, enjoy some of them, and store the remainder. Or you can cook up the Rainbow Vegetables Oven Fries and snack on them.

Pre-make some of your favorites to have on hand when you can't help thinking about the old foods you used to eat, like the burritos or enchilada recipes. Make some and freeze them in case your running late from work and cooking will be just too much to think about. Just warm them up and dinner is served.

Drink water, plain or infused with some lemon or lime. It's refreshing and you're maintaining your hydration.

Eat every three to four hours. When your blood sugar begins to dip is when you feel hunger the strongest. Carry a few MariGold energy bars with you during the day to have on hand, especially during the mid-afternoon when it is usually the time that we feel that blood sugar drop. They especially come in handy if you are on the go for business or travel quite a bit. They are lectin-free and do the trick in maintaining your hunger and cravings.

If you think of food quite often, think of the foods you will now be eating and the necessary condiments, spices, and organic products that you'll need to buy. Distract yourself and do some research as to where the best places are to purchase them and compare pricing either online or at your neighborhood health food market.

Think of some of the recipes you like in this e-book and what you might add as a personal ingredient that will make it all your own. Convert some of the dishes that you liked to eat into lectin-free dishes. Once you get more knowledgeable about ingredients and how they interact with each other, you can even make up your own special recipes.

Research the right kitchen appliances you will need to purchase (if you don't already own them) to make your preparation of the recipes done with ease. And as for the recipes themselves, they are relatively easy to make and are delicious. Remember that many of the measurements of spices and additives you use in the recipes are guides as to how much to use. However, the words "to your taste" mean just that. Taste the food while you're preparing it so when the dish is ready to eat, you will enjoy it more because it is to your taste.

The best advice that anyone can get when they begin to diet and to change the way they prepare and eat food is to think positively, enjoy the 21 days and you'll be happy with the results.

Conclusion

The *Lectin-Free Cookbook: 21 Day Diet Plan To Help You Get Started, Lose Weight and Feel Great - Forty Delicious Plant Paradox Recipes Tips and Tricks for Beginners* is a book that works as a guide to weight loss and healthier eating. It is hoped that you learned more about what it is to be lectin-free, have begun to lose weight and that you enjoyed making and eating some, if not all, of the recipes that were put together to help you reach your goals.

The recipes that have been included in this book are being made by people just like you who had their own health issues to address, or just wanted to adopt a healthier way to eat and found joy in learning how to become a lectin-free convert.

As you know, any diet you choose to follow can be difficult at first. But once you see and feel the difference in how you feel and like what you see in the mirror, you'll be happy that you succeeded in converting to a lectin-free diet. Your family and friends will become curious and ask how you lost the weight or will be amazed that some of the recipes they thought were being made the same old way were actually made with healthy substitutes and are just as flavorful.

Thank you for reading and learning about lectins and lectin-free foods and continue to benefit from this book. If you have a moment, a review on Amazon would be appreciated.

Index

H

Healthy Natural Wraps – Romaine Lettuce and Artichoke Spread

I

Italian Style Mustard Greens and Sweet Potato Soup

L

Leek and Cauliflower Soup
Lectin-Free Chili

M

Macadamia Nuts
Mint Chocolate Cookies
Miso Stir Fry with Mushrooms and Napa Cabbage

N

Nuts as a Snack

O

Orange Cranberry Muffins

P

Pesto & Broccoli with Miracle Noodles
Pine Nuts
Plant Paradox Hemp Seed Protein Smoothie

R

Rainbow Vegetables Oven Fries
Refreshing Citrus Fried Jackfruit Tacos
Rich Dark Chocolate Brownies with Large Sea Salt Flakes

S

Salmon Cakes
Salmon & Orange Salad w. Dijon Vinaigrette
Sea Vegetables Chicken Salad with Miracle Noodles
Snickerdoodle Cookies
Spinach Pesto
Steak & Spinach Salad
Sugar-Free White Chocolate
Sweet Hummus with Roasted Garlic
Sweet Potato Toast

T

Tempeh Bacon & Sweet Potato Breakfast Burritos with
Chipotle Crema
Ten-Minute Avocado Smoothie Bowl
Two-Minute Vanilla Mug Cake

W

Walnuts
Wild Shrimp with Greens & Lemon Oil

Read Others Books From Clarissa Fleming

- Lectin Free Cookbook: 74 Best Easy Lectin-Free Electric Pressure Cooker Recipes: https://www.amazon.com/dp/B07F2KGX94
- Keto Fat Bombs For Lazy People: 38 Must-Try Savory and Sweet Ketogenic Fat Bomb Recipes: https://www.amazon.com/dp/B07K5C4QLJ
- Intermittent Fasting: 5:2 Fast Diet For Beginners: https://www.amazon.com/dp/B07L9BPDKW
- Freestyle 2018: 105 Best Easy And Healthy Recipes To Quickly Lose Weight: https://www.amazon.com/dp/B07HRT1R35
- Lectin Free Cookbook: No Hassle Lectin Free Recipes In 30 Minutes or Less: https://www.amazon.com/dp/B07H7T2SVM

Made in the USA
Middletown, DE
19 July 2019